365 WAYS TO GET FIT

Andrew Shields

in association with

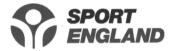
SPORT ENGLAND

COLLINS & BROWN

First published in Great Britain in 2008 by
Collins & Brown
10 Southcombe Street
London W14 0RA

Text copyright © Collins & Brown 2008

Distributed in the United States and
Canada by Sterling Publishing Co,
387 Park Avenue South, New York,
NY 10016, USA

British Library Cataloguing-in-
Publication Data:
A catalogue record for this book is
available from the British Library.

ISBN: 978-1-84340-384-5

Reproduction by Spectrum Colour Ltd, UK

Printed and bound by Craft Print
International Limited, Singapore

Over 50 per cent of England's population
does no sport or physical activity at all.
Sport England's ambition is to change that
and to get 2 million people doing more
sport by 2012.

Sport England aims to make sport and
active recreation easy, convenient and
attractive. Its aim is to help people make
sport part of their day-to-day lives, no
matter how busy their lifestyles might be.

The good news is that building more
activity and sport into your day is easier
than you might think. By taking it one
step at a time and starting small you can
get that bit closer to your goals – getting
fit, losing weight or spending more time
with the kids – whatever they might be.

Your first step might be to play footie
in the park with the family instead of
going to the cinema – it's all about
finding what works for you. By gradually
increasing your amount of activity and
finding the sports that are right for you,
you could become healthier, fitter, lose
some weight or simply have more fun.

This book is full of practical advice
and ideas to help you make those small
changes that can make a big difference.

You can find more ideas and
information on getting active at:
www.sportengland.org/getactive

CONTENTS

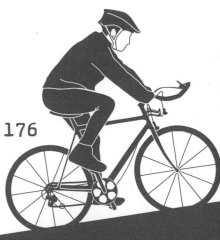

CONGRATULATIONS!

What for, you may be asking. I haven't done anything yet!

Well, simply by picking up this book you've shown that you're interested in becoming more active, and in feeling fitter and healthier. The challenge now is to get out there and do it:

> IT'S A FACT THAT SINCE THE MID-1980s, THE DISTANCE PEOPLE WALK HAS DROPPED BY MORE THAN 20 PER CENT.

> THE DISTANCE PEOPLE CYCLE HAS DROPPED BY 10 PER CENT.

> THE DISTANCE PEOPLE DRIVE HAS RISEN BY 70 PER CENT.

This book is about reversing that trend. It's about building more sport and physical activity into our daily lives. And it's about seeing that activity as an opportunity to make a difference, not as something to be avoided. Otherwise, the alarming rise in obesity, type-2 diabetes, heart disease and chronic conditions associated with a sedentary society will spiral out of control.

Instead of waiting until your body creaks and wheezes to a halt, prevent it from happening by taking responsibility for your health.

SMALL CHANGES CAN MAKE A BIG DIFFERENCE. SO WHAT ARE YOU WAITING FOR?

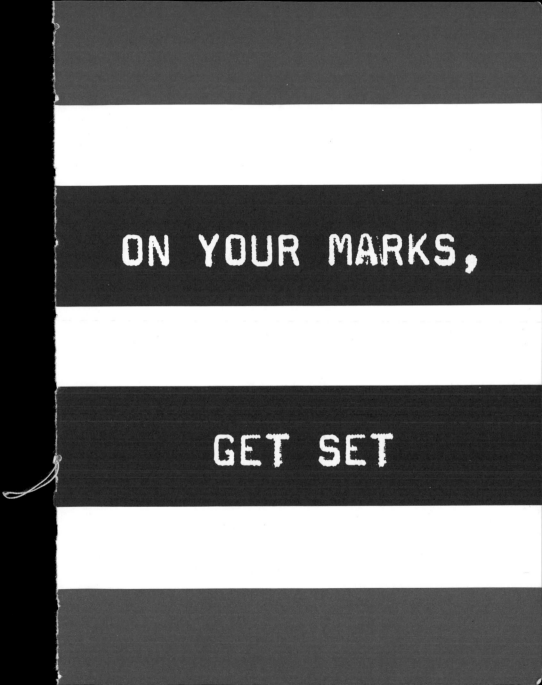

ON YOUR MARKS,

GET SET

HOW ACTIVE ARE YOU NOW?

1. WHERE DO YOU LIVE?

a) In a house with one or more flights of stairs

b) In a ground-floor flat or bungalow

c) In a first-floor (or above) flat – and I usually use the stairs

d) In a first-floor (or above) flat – and I usually use the lift

2. WHAT IS YOUR MAIN MODE OF TRANSPORT?

a) Public transport (bus, train, or tube/metro)

b) Car or motorbike

c) Bicycle

d) Walking

3. FOR HOW LONG WOULD YOU WALK OR CYCLE IN A TYPICAL WORKING DAY?

a) Less than 10 minutes

b) 10–20 minutes

c) 20–30 minutes

d) At least half an hour or more

4. WHAT DO YOU USUALLY DO AT LUNCHTIME?

a) Stay where I am and eat lunch at my desk

b) Go out to buy sandwiches

c) Go for a walk

d) Play sport or exercise

5. AT WORK, HOW DO YOU MOVE FROM FLOOR TO FLOOR?

a) Always take the lift

b) Walk up or down – but only one flight, mind

c) Walk up or down any number of flights

d) We're on the ground floor!

6. DO YOU OWN A DOG?

a) No

b) Yes, and I walk it regularly

c) Yes, and I walk it occasionally

d) Yes, and I employ a dog-walker

7. YOU'VE JUST GOT HOME AND DISCOVER YOU ARE OUT OF MILK. WHAT DO YOU DO?

a) Turn around and walk to the shops

b) Send someone else to get it

c) Drive to the shops

d) Do without

8. HOW DO YOU SHOP?

a) Drive to a supermarket once a week

b) Shop locally more than once a week and carry it home

c) Shop locally more than once a week and drive home

d) Me? Shopping?

9. IF YOU HAD TO RUN 50 METRES FOR A BUS, HOW WOULD YOU FEEL?

a) Barely out of breath

b) I'd be glad to sit down and recover

c) I'd be red in the face and panting for five minutes

d) I'd wait for the next one

10. DO YOU CURRENTLY PLAY A SPORT OR EXERCISE?

a) At least three times a week

b) About once or twice a month

c) Once in a while

d) Never/Not if I can help it

Now turn over to check your scores…

HOW ACTIVE ARE YOU NOW?

ANSWERS

1. a) 4   b) 0   c) 4   d) 0
   (Add one point if you have a garden)
2. a) 3   b) 0   c) 4   d) 4
3. a) 0   b) 1   c) 2   d) 4
4. a) 0   b) 1   c) 3   d) 4
5. a) 0   b) 2   c) 4   d) 0
6. a) 0   b) 4   c) 2   d) 0
7. a) 4   b) 0   c) 0   d) 0
8. a) 0   b) 4   c) 1   d) 0
9. a) 4   b) 2   c) 1   d) 0
10. a) 4   b) 2   c) 1   d) 0

HOW DID YOU SCORE?

30–40: Congratulations! You probably exercise regularly, are active in everyday life, and are well motivated to continue.

20–30: Pretty good: you understand that it's important to exercise and want to find ways to be even more energetic.

10–20: Could do better: you're missing too many opportunities to build physical activity into your daily routine.

0–10: Don't despair! This book is aimed at people just like you, who want to be more active but need help and support to get started.

There are many reasons for a low score. Perhaps it's hard to take a regular break from your job, or a hectic lifestyle makes it impossible to fit in a walk, or the car is your only viable means of getting about. Making the effort to build physical activity into everyday life may seem like too much hard work. But read on – in the 'Go!' section there are dozens of easy, fun ideas to get you started.

TWENTY GREAT REASONS FOR...

1 To cut your risk of coronary heart disease

2 To sleep better

3 To have more energy to play with the kids

4 To give your sex life more oomph

5 To cope better under stress

6 To feel happier

7 To boost your brain power

8 To have fun

9 To walk up a flight of stairs without getting out of breath

10 To make new friends

...GETTING MORE ACTIVE

11 To move without bits of you wobbling

12 To enhance your balance and coordination

13 To give you more confidence

14 To perk up your skin tone

15 To learn new skills

16 To reduce your risk of osteoporosis

17 To improve your circulation

18 To improve your metabolism

19 To slow down the ageing process

20 To feel good about yourself!

WHAT IS FITNESS?

OK! Inspired by those 20 great reasons to get more active, we're raring to go. But what exactly do we mean by 'fitness'?

There are five basic components of fitness, and the aim of our exercise programme is to try and address them all. The five are: cardiovascular fitness, muscular strength, muscular endurance, flexibility and more fitness.

CARDIOVASCULAR FITNESS

Sometimes abbreviated to CV, this is nothing to do with job applications but is about the efficiency of our heart, lungs and circulatory system. It's also known as stamina, endurance or aerobic fitness. Activities which get the heart pumping, such as exercise to music, running, dancing, climbing stairs, cycling, swimming and brisk walking will all boost cardiovascular fitness.

IT MIGHT FEEL LIKE A LOT OF EFFORT TO GET HEALTHY, BUT IT'S A LOT LESS EFFORT THAN WAKING UP ONE DAY WITH TYPE-2 DIABETES.

JAMES CRACKNELL
OLYMPIC ROWER

MUSCULAR STRENGTH

This is the ability of a muscle to exert maximum force against a resistance, and it is just as important for women as for men. By increasing the amount of resistance, we can train our muscles to work more efficiently. Weight training is a great way to increase muscular strength, but it doesn't have to be done in a gym. Carrying bags of shopping home rather than putting them in the boot of the car and driving, digging the garden, and even performing simple exercises with a 1kg (2lb) bag of sugar in each hand will increase muscular strength. And don't worry about going too far – you would have to be very committed and lift very heavy loads indeed to end up looking like Popeye!

MUSCULAR ENDURANCE

When muscles are able to work for a prolonged period of time without fatigue they have good endurance. We often think of endurance as being the preserve of marathon runners and Tour de France cyclists, but we all need good levels of muscular endurance simply to live our lives to the full without feeling exhausted. A long walk or bike ride, for example, will do wonders for muscular endurance in the lower body.

FLEXIBILITY

Our bodies become stiff with lack of use. Muscles, ligaments and tendons that once made it easy to touch our toes become tighter. Sometimes, even everyday movements can be difficult as we literally seize up. Flexibility is the aspect of fitness we most often ignore. However, regular stretching can not only restore suppleness and range of movement, but it can improve it. Stretching also helps to ease tension, tone muscles and has a positive effect on posture.

MOTOR FITNESS

Motor fitness is not about fine-tuning your car, but about fine-tuning your body. It includes agility, balance, coordination, speed, reactions and power – all features that come naturally to great sportsmen and women, but which we lesser mortals can work on and improve as well. Regular exercise will enhance motor fitness alongside the four other components we've just explored.

GO BUDDY GO!

21 **What's the best investment** you can make if you're committed to getting fit?

- A pair of flashy trainers with go-faster stripes?
- Membership of that swish new health club around the corner?
- A new pair of knees?!

In fact one of the biggest assets of all is a friend. A friend who will drag you out of the house when it's raining, when there's something good on the telly or when you've had a hard day at work. Even when there's a bottle of wine in the fridge just asking to be drunk, or you're feeling lazy and unmotivated, a friend who will arrive with a big smile and an intravenous drip full of that completely legal drug called 'enthusiasm'. And, of course, when it's your pal who's making excuses, you'll do exactly the same for them. Won't you? Everyday activity is so much easier when you've got someone to talk to, laugh with, call on and chivvy you along when the going gets tough.

What do you need to get moving? Not very much at all!
Pull on some comfortable clothes and you're all set to go.

22 **If you are going to be running or playing sport, a pair of supportive, cushioned training shoes is essential.** Don't be swayed by how they look or what a persuasive salesperson tells you and instead seek advice from a specialist retailer. Some running shops have scanning machines that will take photos of your feet to ensure a perfect fit. Expect to pay around £50–£70 for specialist running shoes; it will be money well spent.

23 **A pedometer counts your steps and can be a useful way of tracking how far you have walked each day.** You can buy one at most sports stores.

24 **A water bottle.** Too many of us don't drink enough water and the amount you need increases as you exercise. There are specialist top-of-the-range 'hydration systems' on sale but, quite honestly, a filled plastic bottle does the job perfectly if you're going out for a long walk.
Add some squash if you need a little flavour.

25 **The best way to keep track** of your activity levels is to write down what you've done. A notebook is fine; you could open a file on your computer or create your own wall chart. The most important thing is to log your exercise regularly, or you'll forget what you've done.

Make a record of what you did, and for how long. Don't just list sport and exercise, include:

- Housework
- Gardening
- Walking or cycling to and from work
- Shopping
- Playing with the kids
- Anything else that got you moving – such as walking up and down the stairs a dozen times during the day.

If you wear a pedometer, keep a note of the daily distance and total number of steps – then try to beat the figures the next day.

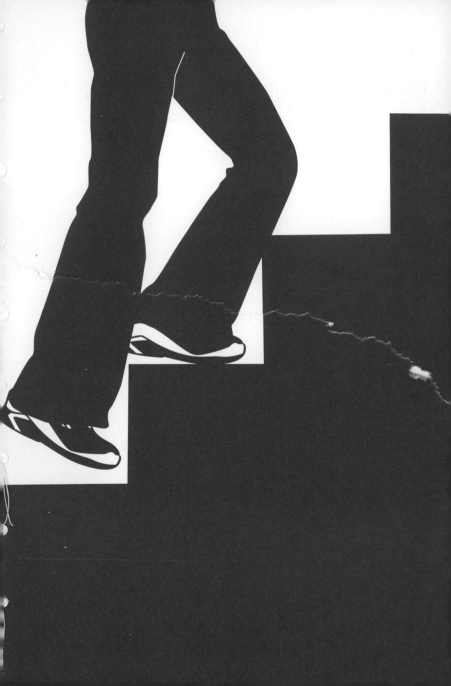

Also write about how you felt during and after the activity: were you full of energy or feeling lethargic? Did you finish your workout with a satisfied smile, or slump into a chair with a yawn?

If you plan to make changes to your diet with the aid of the healthy eating section later in this book, you may want to keep a food diary as well. This is quite time-consuming as you'll need to record everything you eat and drink, together with approximate portion sizes. However, it will give a clear picture of your daily intake – which you can share with your doctor or a qualified nutritionist if you want advice on the way to achieve long-lasting benefits.

Be honest! Or you'll only be cheating yourself.

BE REALISTIC!

26 **How often should you exercise, and for how long?** The answer is simple: try to move your body and be active as often as you can, and for as long as feels comfortable. Your aim is to gradually increase the amount of activity in your life – an extra bike ride here, an additional game of football with the kids there – and to extend the duration. Stay out half an hour longer when walking in the country, or, at the end of an afternoon's gardening session, dig over the flowerbed you were planning to leave until next week.

What you are doing is challenging your body to go beyond its current level of fitness – but doing it gradually. Don't go crazy and start running every day because it is probably unsustainable. If you feel particularly tired take a day off to allow your body to recover.

In this way, small changes you make to your lifestyle will build together to make a big difference.

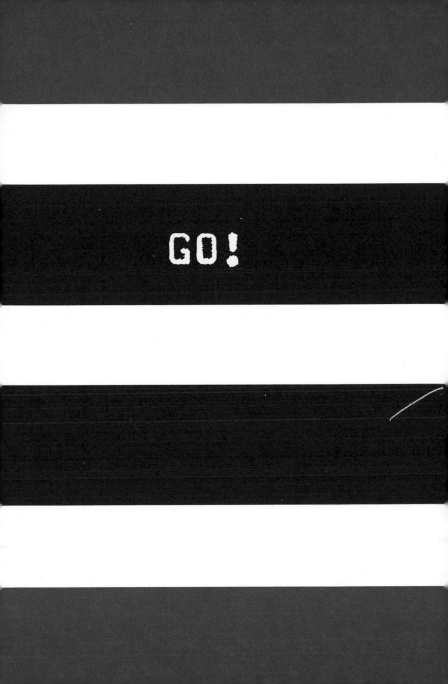

KEEP IT IN THE FAMILY

Research shows that active parents tend to have active children. Kids need role models and none is more powerful than a parent, particularly for girls. If your children see that you value fitness, physical activity and good health, they are more likely to as well.

27 **When there's a birthday party to organise, base it on activity.** If it's a summer celebration, plan a walk and picnic in the country. Swimming, tenpin bowling and multi-sports parties are popular at any time of the year.

28 **If you take your children to a local sports club, why not walk or cycle there rather than driving.** It's a great warm-up for all of them as well as you. When you're there, don't just use their session as a chance to slob out with a book or gossip with other parents. You may not want to play football or tennis, but is there another activity that you fancy? If not, how about a half-hour walk around the grounds – still leaving time for a coffee afterwards?

29 When watching your child playing in a match, you don't have to stand or sit in one place for the duration. You could walk along the touchlines or around the perimeter of the playing area, cheering the players on.

IN THE PARK

30 **Going to the playground?** Release your inner child when you're there with chin-ups and dips on the climbing frame, lunges on the wobbly balance plank (great for core stability), climbing on the monkey bars and, if the swings are strong enough to support an adult's weight, a swing to finish with.

31 **Pushing the kids on the swings** works the triceps and shoulder muscles and enhances flexibility throughout the whole body.

32 **Feed the ducks.** The rotator cuff, a group of four small muscles involved in the rotation of the shoulder, does not get used enough. When you throw bread, it does.

33 **If you're organising a picnic,** don't forget to take a bat and ball. Work up an appetite for lunch with a game of French cricket: the batter is not allowed to move his feet and must twist to hit the ball. If the ball hits his legs, he is out – the bowler bowls at the legs, which acts as the wicket. Any fielder can bowl at the batter.

34 **After lunch, play rounders,** with four coats as bases around which the batter must run. Hit the ball and you've got to run; miss it three times or give a catch and you're out.

35 **Finish off with a game of continuous cricket:** after hitting the ball, the batter must run to a coat or stump placed parallel to the 'wicket', about 7m (23ft), away. The bowler can bowl at the wicket as soon as he or she receives the ball, to try to bowl the batter out.

36 **Play 'beans' with a group of children.** Shout 'Runner bean' and everyone has to run on the spot. 'Broad bean': make a large shape. 'Jelly bean': wobble like a jelly. 'French bean': strike a pose and shout 'Bonjour!'. 'Chilli bean': shiver and shake. Encourage creativity: what would you do on the call of 'Baked bean' or even 'Mr Bean'?

ON TARGET

Target games are not only great fun but a perfect way for the whole family to improve their fitness.

37 **Organise a tenpin bowling trip**. Bowling burns 145 calories per hour. Even small children can play, using a chute to bowl the ball and bumpers to prevent the ball rolling into the gutter. Winner buys the drinks afterwards.

38 **Pétanque?** Ooh, la-la! You can play the game otherwise known as boules in any back garden or park. Make sure you bend ze knees for each shot!

39 **Quoits is a great old-fashioned target game.** If you can't buy a set of quoits, improvise with toy rings and a garden trowel stuck in the ground as the target.

40 **Use your imagination to devise target games:** trying to throw tennis balls into a bucket, or rolling them on to a doormat about 15m (49ft) away, will bring out the competitive streak in all age groups.

FUN AND GAMES

41 **Buy a hula hoop and practise wiggling your waist** to prevent the hoop dropping to the ground. Who's the champion wiggler in your family or group of friends?

42 **Climbing is a fantastic workout for the whole body,** demanding strength, flexibility and coordination. All indoor climbing centres run sessions for beginners and for children, with tuition and equipment provided.

43 **Buy a basketball hoop** for the wall of your house or a freestanding netball ring. As well as practising shooting, you can play games such as parents v kids or boys v girls.

44 **Kids love chasing and bursting bubbles.** Blow them high or low to encourage jumping or bending; the kids have to burst them with heads or hands, or have to lie down and burst them with toes only.

45 **You can have an Easter egg hunt at any time of the year.** Indoors or out, everyone has to chase around trying to be first to find the hidden treats.

46 **Kids love challenges 'against the clock'.** Using a timer or watch with a second hand, see who can run to the end of the garden and back the quickest. Or, who can throw and catch the ball against the wall ten times? Or, who can complete five jumping jacks?

47 **Set fun physical challenges using cards and dice.** Everyone writes a challenge on a piece of card (cartwheel, sit-up, forward roll, and so on); these are then shuffled and placed face-down in a stack. Each player draws a card then rolls the dice – and has to complete that number of cartwheels or whatever.

48 **There's nothing more exhilarating than flying a kite** on a windy day. You'll burn plenty of calories running to get the kite airborne and chasing after it when it crashes! Power kites demand considerable strength and stamina to control.

49 **Spend time with the children making swords from cardboard tubes** – then go out into the garden and stage a medieval sword fight. Old curtains make great cloaks.

50 **Buy a set of juggling balls** and teach yourself to keep all three in the air at one time. Great for coordination, balance and flexibility – and not that difficult. Really!

51 **A game of marbles** in the back yard will get you bending into all sorts of funny positions. Play with a target, like golf, or place all the marbles in a circle except for a shooter. You keep all those your shooter knocks out of the circle. Or make up your own rules.

52 **If you own a PlayStation 2,** use the EyeToy camera to stage family sporting challenges. Surprisingly addictive fun for all ages!

53 **Build a human pyramid** with family and friends. Or work in pairs to create the most interesting shape.

54 **A rebounder (mini-trampoline) is a fantastic fitness investment.** A three-minute bounce will raise the heart rate, improve muscle tone, boost circulation and help with balance. It's low-impact exercise and gentle on the joints. And best of all, it's great fun. Kids love rebounding as much as adults, and it's a great way to disguise exercise as play. Once you've mastered the basic bounce, you can add knee raises, kicks to side and front, jumping jacks, twists and even jogging. Or prepare for a skiing holiday with slalom and downhill movements.

5 5 **You don't need proper equipment to play cricket.**
Scrunch up a sheet of paper and tape it into a
round shape to make a ball. A cardboard tube will do fine for
the bat. And a dustbin makes a perfect wicket. Make up your
own rules: if you're playing in the lounge, a shot under the
bookcase scores four and down the back of the sofa is out!

5 6 **Play 'Traffic Lights'.** Colour three cards: one red,
one amber and one green. Give the cards to the
person who is going to be the traffic warden. Everyone walks
around and when the traffic warden holds up a red card,
turns themselves into a statue. The amber card means that
you have to hop on one leg – waiting for the green card,
when you can race around at top speed. Then change the
traffic warden, vary the commands and add combinations:
green followed by red is usually entertaining.

5 7 **Assign a different fun activity to each room of
your house or flat:** for example, five sit-ups in the
lounge, ten star jumps in the kitchen, five hops on one leg
along the hall, and so on. Get the kids to draw reminder
posters to stick to each door. Every time you enter that room,
you have to do the activity. Try to go a whole day without
forgetting, with everyone checking each other. Afterwards
leave the posters on the doors and aim to do every activity
once, every day.

FUN THINGS TO DO WITH A BALLOON

58 **Play 'keepy-up'.** See who can keep the balloon off the ground for the longest. Try it first with hands, head and feet, then feet only and then, hardest of all, head only.

59 **Play balloon volleyball.** Use a bed or a table as the net. If the balloon hits the floor, it's a point.

60 **Play balloon tennis.** Again, use a bed or a table as the net. Play with plastic rackets – or have fun making some out of corrugated cardboard.

61 **Relive great moments on the football pitch** in slow motion, using a balloon instead of the ball.

62 **Rub a balloon on a sweater to create static electricity** and 'stick' it to the ceiling or a wall. Who can jump highest to retrieve it?

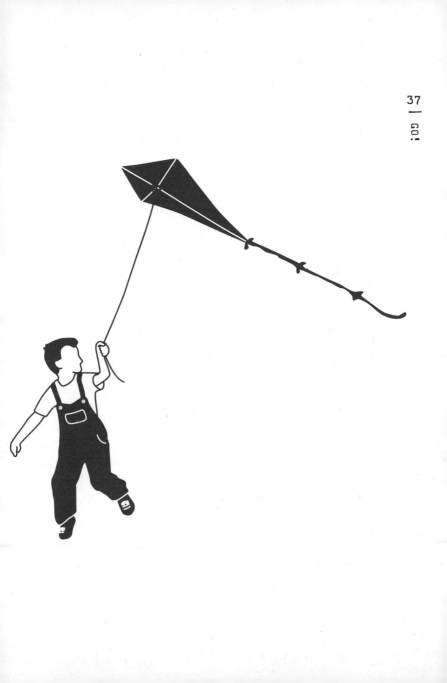

LIFE'S A BEACH

On holiday it's tempting to lie in the sun all day, but a morning or late afternoon walk along the beach with your feet in the sea is enjoyable and invigorating. Remember to wear sunscreen and cover up with clothes if the sun is still hot, and sit in the shade during the hottest part of the day.

Alternatively, why not play a beach game together before running into the sea to cool off.

6 3 **This is a great game for the beach,** or you can play on any hard surface, such as a patio, drive or playground. All you need is a tennis ball.

Mark out a 'court' about 2m x 2m (6ft x 6ft) and divide it into two halves. Player one bounces the ball in her court then palms it over the imaginary net and player two returns it. The aim is to score a point by hitting a shot that your opponent can't return. You score points whether you are serving or receiving. The first one to get ten wins.

You can play singles or doubles, 'winner stays on', or set up a little tournament with family and friends. You can handicap adults by giving children a few points' start or make adults play with their 'wrong' hand. If you don't want to be competitive, see how long you can keep a rally going.

The game will get you stretching and reaching, and it's good for hand-eye coordination. Just like proper tennis, in fact.

FLY A FRISBEE!

64 **Flinging a flying disc isn't just for kids:** even some of Manchester United's stars do it! It's simple, cheap and all you need is some open space. A 70kg (154lbs) man will burn around 250 calories in an hour; 'ultimate frisbee' is also great for boosting flexibility, agility and coordination as you jump to make those snazzy catches.

If you really get into it, ultimate frisbee is also a competitive sport with a World Championship. The team game requires you to pass the disc up the pitch – you can't run with it – to reach the end-zone, as in American Football. To find out more, visit www.whatisultimate.com.

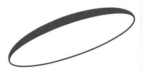

'A VIGOROUS FIVE—MILE
WALK WILL DO MORE GOOD
FOR AN UNHAPPY BUT
OTHERWISE HEALTHY ADULT
THAN ALL THE MEDICINE
AND PSYCHOLOGY IN THE
WORLD.'

DR PAUL DUDLEY WHITE
HEART SPECIALIST, USA

65 **Here's a simple ball game to play with any number of kids.** It will help to sharpen everyone's catching and throwing ability – and their counting skills.

One person is the thrower, and everyone else stands comfortably spaced about 3m (9ft) away. The thrower tosses a ball towards a player and, depending on the difficulty of the throw (and the age and skill of the player), announces a number between 10 and 100, like so: 'I've got 50 points up for grabs.' If the player makes the catch, he gets that number of points. If he drops the ball, though, he loses that number of points.

The first person to get 500 points wins and becomes the thrower for the next game. You can add variations such as altering the distance thrown, catching one-handed, or deducting points for a poor return to the thrower.

THE NUMBERS GAME

66

There are around 210 calories in a can of regular cola.

Try a healthier option or wash them away with:

60 minutes of steady cycling at 10kph (6mph).

40 minutes of tennis.

Or 30 minutes of swimming at two lengths per minute.

There are plenty of other activities you can do at the beach to help burn calories, apart from organised games.

67 **Use a foot pump to blow up inflatables** – this action works and tones the front of the thigh and the bottom muscles.

68 **Can you see another beach?** Check it out by walking to it. What's around the headland? Again, set out on foot for a voyage of discovery.

69 **Use plastic cups to make sand 'tenpins'** – then see who can demolish the most by rolling a tennis ball at them from about 10m (30 feet) away.

70 **On a pebble beach, build a target of four or five stones piled on top of each other.** Each player collects five small stones, retreats 6–7m (19–23ft) and carefully takes pot shots at the target. Whoever knocks the target over wins a point.

71 Waves were surely designed to be jumped over!

72 Build as many sandcastles as you can in 30 minutes.
The race is on! Once you've finished building you can take it in turns to undo all your hard work by demolishing your sandcastles.

73 Sand is great for jumping on. Who's the champion bunny-hopper? Who can travel farthest with ten hops? Use spades, deckchairs and windbreaks to rig up a high jump or hurdles – and keep the entire beach amused watching your antics.

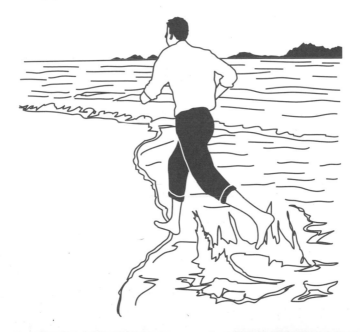

HOT SHOE SHUFFLE

74 TV programmes such as *Strictly Come Dancing* have done wonders for the image of dancing – and have helped thousands of people to discover the delights of moving to music. From ceroc to salsa, ballroom to Bollywood, tap to tango, dancing is not only great fun – it's fantastic exercise as well.

75 Half an hour of ballroom dancing – such as the waltz, tango or quickstep – will burn as many calories as a brisk walk. Even more energetic forms, such as disco and swing, will really improve your aerobic fitness and gobble up to 400 calories in an hour.

76 Dance is a great way to improve balance and coordination – is there a more elegant sight than a couple gliding smoothly across a dancefloor? It also increases muscle tone, bone strength and stamina.

77 **Dance is very sociable.** You need not worry about joining a dance class on your own because teachers usually rotate men and women so that everyone gets a chance to dance with everyone else.

78 **Dance classes have a far lower drop-out rate than gyms,** which many people join but quit within a year because they find that kind of exercise tedious. There's always the challenge of learning new steps to keep you going back week after week.

79 **The easiest way to get your feet moving is to listen to some upbeat music while you're doing domestic chores.** Vacuuming and dusting seem much less dull when you're bopping around the house!

80 **If you'd rather learn a few moves before venturing out to a class, there are plenty of DVDs and videos that will teach you the basics.** Try your local library or video hire store.

You're never too old – or too young – to start dancing. Classes are often advertised in local newspapers, or contact the British Dance Council (www.british-dance-council.org) for details of schools in your area.

WALK THE WALK!

Parents drive an average of 1,000km (600 miles) each year taking their kids to school and back on short, easily walkable journeys. That's two-thirds of the distance from Land's End to John O'Groats...

Inactivity costs the nation an estimated £8 billion a year and if people walked more it could cut this bill.

According to the Environmental Transport Association, car users regularly suffer up to three times as much pollution as pedestrians because they often sit in traffic and the air conditioning sucks in exhaust fumes from the car in front.

81 **The easiest change you can make to your lifestyle is to walk more.** Whether it's to and from work, the shops or school; on your own, with your partner or friends, or as a family, the simple act of putting one foot in front of the other can be a fantastic way to improve your fitness on an everyday basis.

82 **Not only is walking a completely natural activity, it requires no equipment except for comfortable footwear.** It's aerobic because it improves the efficiency of the heart and lungs and, as a low-impact exercise, it places minimal stress on joints and muscles.

83 **Regular walking is great for toning your legs and bum;** it will also lower your resting heart rate and blood pressure. Getting out and about is a superb stress-reliever, no matter whether you're walking in the open countryside or in an urban setting.

84 **A 70kg (154lb) man walking his dog for an hour at a moderate 5kph (3mph) will burn around 250 calories.** If he increases the pace to 7kph (4mph) that number will rise to 300. Add some hills to climb and he could expend more than 500 calories in an hour of very satisfying activity!

85 **Research has also shown that in terms of cardio-vascular benefits, it's not how hard you exercise but the amount you do that matters.** In an American study, a group of people who jogged 20km (12 miles) per week didn't gain any more cardio benefits than those who walked the same distance in a week.

86 **The key is to walk briskly rather than dawdle.**
Swing your arms to establish a rhythm as you stride out, pushing off from your heels and through your toes, and try to breathe deeply and regularly. Walk tall! Don't slouch or stuff your hands in your pockets. You may want to listen to music as you walk, but don't let it distract you from thinking about your technique – and always be aware of your surroundings and personal safety.

87 **A pedometer** (see page 21) is the most accurate way to measure the distance you walk each day. The most commonly used guideline to aim for is 10,000 steps a day. You may be pleasantly surprised when you first measure your daily distance and record it in your activity diary – or you may be shocked at the meagre step count and forced to recognise just how long you spend sitting at the wheel of a car or behind a desk.

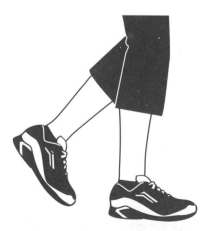

THE NUMBERS GAME

88

A brisk 1.6km (1 mile) walk in 20 minutes burns around 100 calories.

That's as many calories as:

Swimming for 10 minutes.

Playing football for 12 minutes.

Or doing aerobics for 16 minutes.

89 **Get off the bus one stop early** and you'll burn six calories for each minute that you walk.

90 **Go through regular doors rather than the automatic ones.** Pushing a door recruits your triceps (back of the arms), shoulders and chest muscles.

91 **Carry paper and bottles to the recycling station.** Every minute you walk will burn six calories – far more if the load is heavy.

92 **A dog is an ideal aid to fitness.** Keeping a dog to heel on its lead adds slightly to the six calories per minute required for walking. Researchers in Canada found that dog owners walked for an average of five hours per week compared to less than three hours for the pooch-less. If you're planning to buy a dog, think big. A chihuahua will be tired out long before you are…

93 **If you like dogs,** become your neighbourhood dog walker. You can walk several dogs at once, and you might even get paid for doing so.

94 **Carry your baby in a sling or backpack** – you will burn around 20 per cent more calories than using a pushchair or a jogger buggy. The core muscles around your lower spine are recruited, too, in order for you to remain firmly upright.

95 **Walk down escalators rather than standing still** – this burns four calories per minute, a figure that increases if you 'put the brakes on', lowering your legs more slowly.

96 **Walking up escalators is a good form of resistance work,** which burns around ten calories per minute. If you go up two steps at a time it's particularly good for the gluteal muscles of your bottom.

97 **Always use the stairs instead of the lift.** As well as burning ten calories per minute, you will work your abductor muscles at the side of the thighs when you turn on to a landing at the top of a flight of stairs.

98 **'Dodge-walk' by sidestepping passers-by.** This burns six calories per minute, and recruits the abductor and adductor muscles of the outer and inner thigh, plus the calves as opposed to linear walking.

99 **Walk off-road** – harder surfaces instantly 'return' energy to the feet whereas, softer surfaces do not, making walking harder.

A relatively active person will walk around 10,000 steps in a day; this should become your intermediate target. You may have to build up to this figure, but you will be surprised by how small things, such as getting off the bus a stop early or walking to the local shop, will make a difference. If you choose to walk further than 10,000 steps it is up to you – but be warned, once you've started it can become addictive and using a pedometer particularly so. You'll soon be taking a longer way home just to get those numbers up!

100 **Around 15,000 women and a few brave men don decorated bras each year to powerwalk a half- or full marathon around London through the night.** The Playtex Moonwalk has so far raised more than £20 million for breast cancer research and is a fabulously empowering event. There are plenty of other events at which you can powerwalk, and full details are at www.walkthewalk.org.

101 **If you don't want to expose your under-wear in public,** the website www.walkingworld.com has a database of more than 3,000 walks of varying distances and degrees of difficulty. You can download full details of a walk for just £1.50.

102 If you like getting out into the countryside, why not join a ramblers' club? The name

may conjure up images of brogues and deerstalker hats, but clubs are simply groups of like-minded people who enjoy a good walk and fresh air. The Ramblers' Association (www.ramblers.org.uk) is an excellent source of information whether you want to walk for health, join a club or get your kids out of the house with you. You can also download the Association's *Take 30* booklet, which includes a ten-week walking plan. The '30', by the way, refers to the 30 minutes of brisk walking we should all accumulate on most, and preferably all, days of the week.

103 Have baby; can exercise! It's sometimes hard finding time to be active when there's an

addition to the family – but in 'powerpramming', baby definitely comes too. Whether it's pushing the pram as a pulse-raiser or holding your newborn to add resistance to squats, a powerpramming workout adds purpose to that daily push around the park. It's sociable, too, as you get to meet other new parents.

To find out more, click on www.powerpramming.co.uk. If there isn't a class in your area, why not ask a qualified fitness instructor at your local gym or sports centre to set up a group? Or just get together with other parents for regular walks in the park.

GOOD SPORTS!

ORIENTEERING

104 **Orienteering is the art of navigating round a course in the shortest possible time using a map.** Some people say that it's like doing *The Times* crossword while out on a jog. There are dozens of 'permanent' courses in parks around Britain where you can get the hang of things, many of which are buggy-friendly. You don't need to run – many people stroll along, on their own, as a couple or as a family. You simply buy a map and information pack from a local sales point then head off the beaten track at a time that's convenient to you. No specialist equipment is needed.

If you want to test your skills at a local event, you'll find colour-coded courses to suit different skill levels, perhaps a special route for young children, and a warm welcome – orienteering is a sociable and family-friendly sport.

For information about the sport and a guide to permanent courses, contact the British Orienteering Federation www.britishorienteering.org.uk.

105

Though it has the image of being a sport for older people, a glance at the leading players taking part in a top televised tournament will show that bowls is genuinely for all ages. There's some gentle bending, walking and carrying involved; your skill at sending the 'woods' on a curving path towards the 'jack' – the nearest wins – will improve with practice. There are more than 2,700 clubs in towns, villages and parks around the country, many of which play on summer weekdays as well as at weekends. In the winter, the sport moves indoors and into purpose-built bowling centres.

All you need to get started is a pair of flat shoes; you can usually hire a set of woods, and most clubs will offer some basic coaching. To find out more, contact the English Bowling Association (www.bowlsengland.com).

TABLE TENNIS

106 **The second biggest participation sport in the world (after football) is growing in popularity in Britain.** It's an immensely skilful and tactical game at the highest level, but the basic technique of looping the small white ball over the net is relatively easy to master. You'll be surprised by how energetic table tennis can be, too, as it involves lots of movement and directional changes around the table.

Just about every sports centre will have some table tennis tables that you can hire for an hour or two, either as a couple or as a family. Alternatively, why not gather a group of friends or workmates together and organise a fun singles or doubles tournament? Buy a small trophy to present to the winner – that will ensure you return to play again!

There are hundreds of table tennis clubs around Britain if you want to take things further. The English Table Tennis Association (www.englishtabletennis.org.uk) will point you in the right direction.

BADMINTON

107 **Virtually every sports centre has badminton courts marked out on the floor** – and you can often hire rackets and a shuttlecock to play this deft, dynamic sport. It demands excellent hand-eye coordination to play well, and top-level players are immensely fit and flexible. However, the shuttle moves slowly enough for most of us to enjoy a casual knock-up, and it's a great game to play as a family or in a mixed group.

Ask at your local sports centre for information about booking a court. You will probably find a club based there as well, should you want to play more regularly or receive some coaching. Contact Badminton England (www.badmintonengland.co.uk) for further details about the sport or to find your nearest club.

INLINE SKATING

108 **Not only is inline skating a terrific whole-body, low-impact exercise for all ages,** for some people it has become a viable form of transport. While others are boiling in traffic jams, the skater can glide past on the pavement looking – and staying – ultra-cool.

Some of us are blessed with perfect balance and a sense of adventure, and can get up and be moving around on eight wheels with ease, but for others booking a course of lessons is a good idea. As well as a pair of skates, you will also need to invest in a protective helmet, wrist, elbow and knee pads – though you may be able to hire or borrow these until you're certain that 'inlining' is for you.

You'll learn the basics of moving forwards and backwards and, crucially, how to stop – as well as mastering the moves that make skating such fashionable fun. Mass skating events are now organised in many cities, when you can join the throng in a marshalled scoot around the streets accompanied by a sound system.

The UK Inline Skating Association (www.ukisa.org) is the body to contact if you want to find out about instruction and good, safe places to skate.

109 **You don't need to be a member of a club or have a handicap certificate to enjoy golf.**
A driving range is just the place to improve your hand-eye coordination and develop flexibility and stamina. Many centres also have computer-guided games to test your distance and accuracy, and will provide small-sized equipment for children.

110 **Everyone can play pitch and putt** – a fun family outing where even the wildest 'thwacker' can sometimes complete a hole in one.

111 **How about a round of crazy golf?** You'll find courses springing up all over the country and not just at seaside resorts. When you're trying to manoeuvre the ball around a windmill or over a bridge, it's sometimes better to be a bad golfer!

112 **Play your own game of 'golf' in a park.** All you need is a frisbee and instead of 18 holes, use 18 trees as targets and count how many shots you take to hit them.

113 **Buy a pair of boxing gloves and a punching ball.** They're great for taking out your frustrations after a tough day at work – and an excellent workout for boosting strength, stamina, flexibility and coordination.

114 **Children love to play-fight,** so let them wear the gloves and pretend to land some blows. Mark out the corners of a ring using socks and, if you've got the *Rocky* CD, put on the theme tune.

115 **Kids also love wrestling with mum and dad.** Not only is it exhausting, it's also great for family bonding.

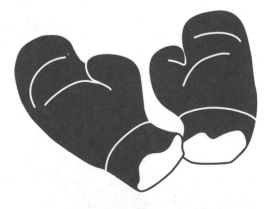

SOME OTHER SPORTS YOU MIGHT NOT HAVE THOUGHT OF...

116 **Triathlon** – A 'Sprint' triathlon – 750m (½ mile) swim, 20km (12 mile) bike ride, 5km (3 mile) run – is a very accessible way to get started in this sport (www.britishtriathlon.org).

117 **Baseball** – Not just for Americans – teams around the country welcome players of all nationalities (www.baseballsoftballuk.com).

118 **Sailing** – Learn the basics in a dinghy before you think of emulating Ellen McArthur! For information, see www.rya.org.uk.

119 **Softball** – A softball is larger and heavier than a baseball and the pitching is done underarm, making this a really fun and sociable sport (www.baseballsoftballuk.com).

120 **Sub-aqua** – Once you've learned to dive safely in a swimming pool you can start to explore exotic locations all over the world (www.bsac.com).

121 **Basketball** – Put a hoop on the side of your house and challenge friends and family to a shootout, or join in a local pick-up game – contact the council to find the nearest court (www.englandbasketball.co.uk).

122 **Korfball** – Similar to basketball and netball but with one key difference: it's a genuinely mixed-sex game. As the old korfball joke goes, you can only mark players of the same sex but you can make a pass at anyone (www.korfball.co.uk).

123 **Netball** – 'Social leagues' have helped to revitalise this women's game, so there's a chance to get involved even if you haven't played since you were at school (www.england-netball.co.uk).

124 **Judo** – Grappling and throwing are the essentials of this Olympic martial art which is fantastic for flexibility, strength and aerobic fitness (www.britishjudo.org.uk).

125 **Volleyball** – This fun sport has been given a boost by the development of 'park volleyball', which is designed for everyone to join in (www.volleyballengland.org).

126 **Windsurfing** – You might start by spending more time in the water than on it, but soon you'll be skimming along (www.rya.org.uk).

127 **Archery** – Whether shooting at a single target or walking through woodland aiming at a variety of targets, such as pictures of animals, archery demands concentration, coordination and stamina (www.gnas.org).

128 **Australian Rules Football** – Fast, physical and skilful, with a great social side. What's more, you don't have to be an Aussie to get involved (www.barfl.co.uk).

129 **Aikido** – This increasingly popular Japanese martial art is designed to turn an aggressor's energy back on himself (www.bafonline.org.uk).

130 **Rowing** – Rowing develops all the main components of fitness. Most clubs run sessions for first-timers (www.ara-rowing.org).

131 **Climbing** – No need to go to the Alps to climb: many sports centres have walls where you can learn the basics (www.thebmc.co.uk).

132 **Squash** – Try this energetic sport by booking a court and hiring rackets at your local sports centre (www.squash.org).

133 **Croquet** – Despite its image as a gentle vicarage tea party pursuit, croquet is a sport of skill and tactical cunning (www.croquet.org.uk).

134 **Wakeboarding** – Like snowboarding on water, and you don't need a speedboat to tow you along (www.britishwaterski.co.uk).

135 **Hockey** – Many clubs run mixed-sex, 'veterans' and social teams where the emphasis is less on winning and more on enjoying a runaround (www.englandhockey.co.uk).

136 **Clay pigeon shooting** – Taking aim at chalk discs simulating the movements of animals and birds requires skill and stamina; it is also very addictive (www.cpsa.co.uk).

137 **Canoeing** – You can learn how to paddle in a swimming pool before venturing on to a river or lake (www.bcu.org.uk).

HOME SWEET HOME

If you're new to exercise and don't wish to go out running or swimming, at least not to start with, or you suffer from an illness or incapacity which makes it difficult to leave your house, don't despair. There are literally hundreds of ways to get active without leaving home.

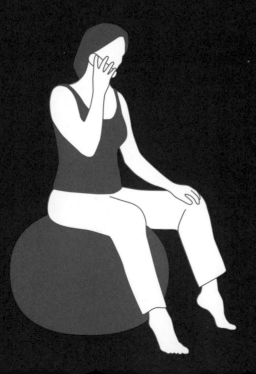

138 **Ditch the TV remote control** – getting up and changing the channel manually ten times a day, with the TV 2m (6ft) from the sofa, will burn an extra ten calories per day. That's a total of 3,650 per year – enough to burn 0.5kg (1lb) of body fat.

139 **When you're watching TV, sit on a fitball rather than slumping in an armchair.** This requires you to use your core stability muscles, which will improve your posture and help to make your abs flatter.

140 **Move around during the ad breaks.** Use the gaps between programmes to walk around – and burn up six calories per minute.

141 **Do your children own a dance mat?** Adults can have fun on them, too. Not only will you burn calories, you can also brush up your dance skills.

142 **After you've read the newspaper, crumple up each sheet.** This works the muscles of your fingers and wrists, and helps to prevent carpal tunnel syndrome, in which pressure increases on the nerves between the hand and wrist.

143 When you've crumpled the sheets of newspaper, press them all together into a big ball. This is an isometric contraction that will exercise the muscles of your shoulders and arms.

144 Now walk with the ball of newspaper to your recycling bin!

145 When sitting, occasionally lift your feet from the floor and hold the position. This works the abdominal and hip flexor muscles.

146 Don't have a newspaper delivered: walk to the local shop and collect it yourself.

147 Is there a gap between two TV programmes you wanted to watch? Don't be tempted to channel-surf to fill the interval: switch the set off and go for a walk. In the half-hour between a soap finishing and the news starting, a 54kg (120lb) woman walking at a steady 6.4kph (4mph) would burn 140 calories.

148 **You know those home workout videos you bought but never looked at?** Well, why not dig them out now? The older and cheesier the better – and if you've still got a pair of stripy legwarmers lurking at the back of the wardrobe, put them on and have some fun.

149 **Fidget!** Squirming around in your seat, standing up and sitting down, and crossing and uncrossing your legs may be irritating if you're at a dinner party, but a persistent fidgeter can, incredibly, burn up to 350 calories per day.

150 **Which sporting events do you really enjoy watching on TV?** If you never miss a rally during Wimbledon, why not find out where your local club is and book a lesson with a coach?

THE NUMBERS GAME

151

Did that pecan Danish pastry go down a treat?

You can burn off the 287 calories you've consumed with:

90 minutes of light housework.

40 minutes of skipping.

Or 25 minutes of steady running at 8kph (5mph).

152 **A garden not only gives you pleasant surroundings in which to relax and a supply of the freshest vegetables and fruit possible, but gardening is also a good workout.** A 70kg (154 lb) man can burn around 350 calories raking, mowing and digging, while these tasks are also great for toning the muscles of the legs, back, abdominals, shoulders and arms. An even better reason for attacking that mossy lawn with gusto!

153 **If you're pruning a tree, chop up the branches.** This is the original core stability exercise, building strength in the deep-set muscles that 'girdle' the spine and are vital for good posture and flat abs.

154 **An hour of vigorous digging, lopping and weeding can burn up to 500 calories.**

155 **Use a watering can rather than a sprinkler** and burn an extra 2 calories per minute for the walking.

156 **Mow the lawn with a traditional mower rather than a powered version.** As well as it burning around 160 calories in 20 minutes, all your main muscle groups will get a workout.

157 **If you don't have a garden, why not rent a plot in an allotment** – and enjoy fresh food, fresh air and plenty of exercise.

158 **Skipping is fantastic cardiovascular exercise,** burning up to 400 calories an hour and boosting your balance, coordination and lightness of movement. So grab that rope from the kids' toybox, head out to the garden and jump to it.

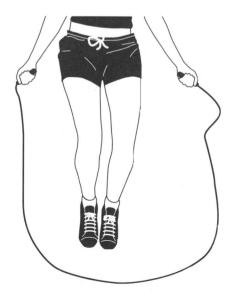

159 **Waiting for the kettle to boil?** Instead of staring out of the window, use those few minutes to tone your chest, shoulders and arms with some press-ups against the kitchen wall. Stand facing the wall with your feet about 90cm (35in) away from it, then reach forward and place your palms on the wall at shoulder height. Carefully lower your body towards the wall, keeping your back straight, and use your arms to control the movement. Tucking your elbows in will target the tricep muscles at the back of the arms. Try to do ten slow repetitions. Then do another ten while the tea brews!

160 **Don't buy ready-chopped vegetables: prepare them yourself.** This uses around two calories per minute, while the washing or scrubbing is of similar benefit.

161 **Use a spoon to mix ingredients instead of an electric whisk** – this uses four calories per minute and works the wrist flexor muscles.

162 **Use your loaf and ditch the bread-making machine.** Kneading dough is a good workout for the arm and chest muscles.

163 **When putting food away after a shopping trip, think of it as a gentle weight-training session.** Do five shoulder presses with the bottle of water before stowing it on the top shelf, and five bicep curls with the bag of potatoes.

164 **Opt for a traditional tin opener rather than an electric version.** As with removing tops from bottles, this exercises the muscles of the forearm and wrist.

165 **Don't use a juicing machine to make a drink:** hand-squeeze the fruit yourself. This is good for the wrist and forearm muscles.

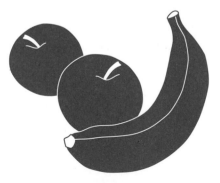

166 **Housework: ugh!** Dusting, vacuuming and cleaning may seem a chore, but it's less boring if you think of the positive impact each stretch, bend, push and pull is having on your body. The movements involved in making a bed can burn around 230 calories an hour, so imagine what washing the kitchen floor can do. What's more, a study has shown that doing household chores can also significantly lower your blood pressure.

167 **Don't skimp on dusting** – with the stretching and walking involved, up to nine extra calories per minute can be burned.

168 **Sweep the path or patio regularly** – it's a good workout for your arms, shoulders and abdominal muscles.

169 **When cleaning, alternate between hands to give both wrists and arms an equal workout.**

170 **Try to get the whole family involved in a spring clean,** or tidying the garage or loft, by offering a treat at the end. Everyone gets a good workout and a reward at the end.

171 **Wash the windows yourself.** Not only do they look good when clean, but it's an activity that uses your arm and shoulder muscles and burns 60 calories in 15 minutes of vigorous rubbing.

172 **Don't spin clothes in the washing machine,** wring them out instead – it's a fantastic workout for the forearms.

173 **Hand-dry clothes** rather than use a tumble drier – a gentle workout for the biceps, front shoulder muscles and chest.

174 **Fifteen minutes of vacuuming** burns around 80 calories and recruits your core stability muscles to maintain good posture.

175 **Give rugs and mats a good beating** – you'll burn around 40 calories in ten minutes and your external obliques (where love handles grow) will get a good workout.

176 **Give the bath a regular clean** even if you're a shower person. A five-minute scrub will burn around 20 calories.

177 **Do the washing-up yourself,** don't use a dishwasher – and reckon on using two extra calories per minute.

178 **When you've washed up the dishes, dry them instead of leaving them to drain** – and count on burning two additional calories per minute.

179 **Put the dishes away one at a time.** Turn your body from side to side, allowing your torso to twist and give a satisfying stretch through the spine.

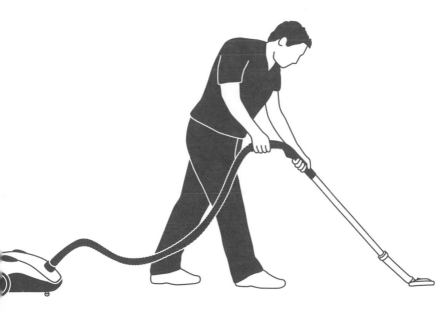

180 **Wash the car instead of using the carwash.** The carwash may be convenient, but you can save money (and water) and burn around 300 calories by giving some TLC to your motor. Don't forget to buff up the bonnet and bumpers to give your arms, shoulders and back muscles a decent workout.

181 **Use good old-fashioned elbow grease** rather than a host of wonder products for polishing. The saw-type motion is great for toning the upper back and shoulder muscles.

182 **Use a traditional dustpan and brush** to clean those difficult corners and help to increase your flexibility.

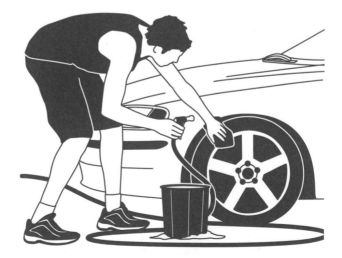

183 **Have more sex!** For a 76kg (168lb) man, 30 minutes of passion burns around 160 calories.

184 **Try not to have too little or too much sleep.** Sleeping for the right amount of time (typically 7–8 hours) means that the body releases sufficient growth hormones, which help to maintain muscle and burn fat. Over-sleeping can result in lower back pain as the body is inactive for too long (especially if your bed is too soft). It also leaves less time for those calorie-burning activities!

185 **If you have a bed with a ladder up to it,** alternate between climbing up the ladder and hauling yourself up. The former works all the leg muscle groups, while the latter works many of the muscles in the back and arms.

186 **Men: alternate between using urinals and sit-down toilets.** Sitting down and then standing up works the muscles in your thighs, bottom and lower back.

187 **Shave your head** – then your body will have to use calories to generate more of its own heat. Regular head shaving will also do wonders for flexibility in your arms and shoulders.

188 **Use a manual toothbrush** – your wrist muscles have to work harder with a manual model than an electric one.

189 **Shower, don't bathe.** Simply standing up uses 0.3 calories per minute, while showering tends to be a more active method of cleaning ourselves than luxuriating in the bath.

190 **Towel your hair dry instead of using a hairdryer.** This provides a gentle workout for the biceps and shoulder muscles, and is also a great stretch for the neck.

191 **Use a razor rather than an electric shaver.** It takes that bit longer and requires greater control from your fingers.

192 **Use roll-on deodorant rather than a spray** – it works the flexor and extensor muscles in the wrist.

193 **Use the upstairs loo** rather than the downstairs one.

194 **After a shower or bath, stretch the backs of your arms** by holding a small towel in your right hand above your head, then grab the other end with your left hand behind your back. Hold for ten seconds, and change sides. Now towel yourself dry.

195 **If you're tiling, cut the tiles yourself.** Using a tile cutter is a good grip-strength workout.

196 **Don't employ someone to paint your hallway.** Climbing up and down the ladder, plus the static contraction at the shoulder joints during the overhead sections, results in around nine calories being burned per minute. And it's cheaper!

197 **Ditch the power tools.** Using a regular screwdriver gives your wrist a workout, and the muscles of the upper arm are used to apply pressure.

198 **Buy flatpack furniture** – carrying and assembling it yourself uses far more energy than waiting for someone to deliver it ready-made. Hammering is particularly good for your shoulders and arms.

199 **Polish your shoes more often** – it's a gentle workout for the shoulders, arms and wrists.

200 **Carefully 'kick' the light switches off.** Lift the knee first, then extend your bare foot so that your toes push the switch. This is beneficial for your thigh and core stability muscles.

201 **Open the garage doors manually.** Getting out of the car, raising the door and returning to the car rather than using a remote control will burn an seven calories per minute.

202 **Always stand rather than sit to do the ironing** – and give the gluteal muscles a workout by clenching and unclenching your buttocks as you work.

203 **Use a doorway to help tone the sides of your shoulders.** Standing upright with your arms hanging straight down, push outwards against the door jambs with the backs of your palms. Hold for 60 seconds then step away from the door, relaxing your arms and letting them drop to your sides. Feel them 'levitate'!

204 **Make hanging out the washing into a workout.** Bend to the basket to collect each item of clothing, give it a vigorous shake and then reach up to the clothes line.

205 **Don't leave cardboard boxes intact for the recycling van to collect** – rip them up first. Tearing corrugated cardboard is especially good for the muscles in the upper and middle back, shoulders and arms.

206 **If you have a loft conversion, visit it regularly** – and use ten calories per minute for climbing the stairs, and four calories per minute coming down them.

207 **Don't spray flies: swat them.** You'll use the rotator cuff muscles in your shoulder to do this, and most other muscle groups as you chase them!

208 **Use a wind-up radio** – every 45 minutes you'll have to walk over to it and wind it up, burning calories and working the wrist and forearm muscles.

209 **Crush tins by foot or hand** before taking them to be recycled – working the front of the thighs, or the forearm muscles.

210 **When moving furniture, lift in the style of a 'dead lift',** with thighs parallel to the floor and back strong throughout, before straightening your legs and pushing your hips forward. In this way, your shoulders, upper and lower back, thighs and calves are all recruited – and you will lift without danger of injury.

211 **Open doors from near the hinge side.** This requires a brief, intense muscular contraction from your triceps, shoulders and chest.

212 **Slowly raise and lower the blinds** – the muscles of your upper back are recruited on the raising phase, while the front of the shoulders come into play during lowering. The core muscles around your lower spine will keep you stable throughout.

213 **Wear less!** By doing so you'll have to create your own body heat, which is the very root of the calorific process (one calorie being the amount of heat required to raise the temperature of one gram of water by one degree Celsius).

214 **Turn down the heating** in your home or office and, by doing so, turn up your body's inner furnace, thereby burning more calories.

215 **Check your posture regularly** – chin in, chest out, shoulders relaxed, back tall, stomach in. Slouching will make your gut appear bigger and can cause pain in the lower back.

216 **Use bottles rather than cans** – prising off bottle tops provides a gentle workout for the muscles that turn the palm upwards and downwards.

217 **Buy a wind-up watch,** which requires you to use the joints of your thumb.

218 **If you enjoy a candlelit atmosphere,** remember to blow out the candles from a distance – a good way to expel any build-up of unwanted carbon dioxide in your lungs.

219 **Wear lace-up shoes** rather than slip-ons – tying them works the thumb and finger flexor muscles. And when they need refastening, your leg muscles are recruited as you bend.

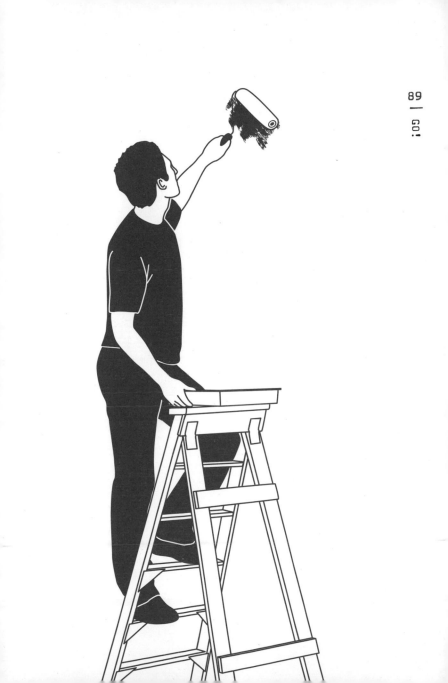

220 **Don't wear a hat.** Since much heat leaves the body via the head, going hatless means your metabolism will keep having to be cranked up to keep you warm.

221 **Be mobile on your mobile** – burn six calories per minute walking while talking, rather than standing still.

222 **If you're a regular visitor to a fitness centre** but, like many, focus solely on weight-training exercises when you get there, add a cardiovascular workout by ditching the car and walking to and from the gym.

223 **Carry objects at arm's length.** Keeping your arms fully extended requires a powerful static contraction of your shoulders and chest muscles, and is also good for your abs.

Even if you're in what might be considered the unhealthy environment of the pub, you can still take opportunities to improve your fitness.

224 **Help carry the drinks from the bar** even if it's not your round, and burn six calories per minute. Raising yourself from your seat will work all the muscle groups in your legs.

225 **Play a few games of darts** – and boost your hand-eye coordination as well as enjoying the calorie-burning effect of walking to and from the board.

226 **A game of snooker or pool** will get you bending over the table to line up and make each shot, boosting your flexibility.

227 Carry a basket instead of using a trolley at the supermarket. This recruits the shoulder, upper and lower arm muscles, and challenges your core stability.

228 Carry your goods home in evenly weighted bags rather than shoving them in the boot of the car.

229 Make frequent walking trips to the supermarket and try to restrict visits by car. You'll burn 200 calories for every mile that you walk.

230 Be forgetful! If you always have to 'go back to get something', you'll burn six calories per minute during the walk.

FOOD AND DRINK

231 **Use self-service cafés when you can.** The walk to the counter, stretching for your plate, walking along the counter and then to a table all adds up, plus you achieve mild toning for your arms and core stability muscles when you carry the tray.

232 **Visit a 'pick your own' fruit farm.** In addition to collecting wonderfully fresh and nutritious food, the further you stretch your arms when picking, the more work your triceps and shoulders are required to do. The lower the fruit, the more your abdominal muscles are recruited.

233 **Drink plenty of water with meals.** This helps you to feel full, eat less and avoid adding unnecessary calories.

TRAIN ON THE TRAIN

Using transport doesn't have to involve sitting still and waiting for the bus/train to reach your destination. Make use of the time to improve your fitness.

234 **Stand rather than sit when travelling on public transport,** and attempt to balance without holding on tightly to a strap or handrail. Just 'roll' with the movement. This is a good workout for the core stability muscles that girdle your lower spine, and can help to prevent lower back pain.

235 **On the bus, always climb up to the top deck** – a good, intense workout for your legs.

236 **Pace up and down the platform when the train is late** and you'll burn six calories per minute.

237 Use a small-wheeled, collapsible bike to commute. A regular-sized bike, ridden at 18kph (12mph), burns nine calories per minute. A small-wheeled bike requires more effort from the riders; you also benefit from folding and carrying it.

238 Don't wait for the bus: stride out to the next stop – six calories are burned for every minute walked, plus you gain a gentle workout for the core stability muscles and the external obliques (sides of the abs) when you twist round to see where the bus is. And maybe you can add in a sprint when it arrives!

239 If you have to drive, park at the top of the multi-storey car park, then walk down the stairs (four calories per minute) and back up again later (ten calories per minute).

240 On an aeroplane, walk up and down the aisle regularly and move your legs while sitting. Such simple exercises can alleviate the danger of deep-vein thrombosis (DVT).

241 When the traffic lights are red, pull in your tummy muscles and clench your buttocks. Hold until the lights turn green! Great for firming your bottom.

EASY DOES IT

242 **Yoga** – Most of us try yoga as a way to chill out and de-stress. However, it's also fantastic for developing flexibility, stamina and strength, while boosting balance and coordination. Research also shows that regular yoga can increase bone density, thus helping to prevent osteoporosis.

There are lots of different styles of yoga, but all are developments of hatha yoga, which is the type you're most likely to come across in a local class. The pace is slow, making it good for beginners, and there's an emphasis on breathing, relaxation and postures known as asanas. You may also come across astanga yoga, which links postures together into a constant flow of movement, which can be fast and challenging with an intense, dynamic breathing technique.

Iyengar yoga, meanwhile, is a very controlled form in which the emphasis is on getting the detail of every posture correct, and can be beneficial for anyone suffering from back pain.

Bikram or 'hot' yoga is currently very fashionable. It involves performing a sequence of 26 postures in a room heated to 37°C (108°F). This allows the muscles to stretch and maximises regeneration of the body, though it's certainly not to everyone's taste.

The best source of information is the British Wheel of Yoga (www.bwy.org.uk), which maintains a directory of trained instructors. However, word of mouth and the noticeboard in your local library, café or wholefood store are also good ways to find out who's teaching in your area. You don't need any special clothing, though you may want to buy your own yoga mat.

One word of caution: yoga, like tai chi and Pilates, will not help you lose weight because for the vast majority of us it is not a cardiovascular activity. Combine it with something like swimming, dancing or cycling, though, and you've got a great exercise package.

243 **Tai chi** – Few activities are as graceful and meditative as tai chi, best known from the BBC 'ident' featuring a group of practitioners dressed in loose red clothing slowly waving their arms and balancing on one leg. Its gentle, flowing movements are relaxing and elegant to perform, leaving students feeling rooted to the earth like a mountain with their heads suspended from the sky by a golden thread.

Tai chi is a holistic approach to fitness and well-being, based on the ancient Chinese philosophy of yin and yang – natural forces that interchange in a seemingly chaotic but always balanced way. Tai chi can reduce stress by calming the mind, body and soul, while the movements undertaken stimulate the flow of 'chi' energy through the body. Its effect on conditions such as circulatory problems, insomnia, back pain and rheumatism are well documented, while several studies have shown its benefits for people of all ages, particularly in keeping us supple, mobile and confident on our feet.

There are tai chi schools throughout Britain, and you will find beginners' classes in community and sports centres, and on adult education programmes. These will teach a 'form', a continuous sequence of movements involving 24, 48 (short forms) or 108 (long form) steps. You don't need any special equipment other than loose-fitting clothes and flat shoes. Although tai chi can take years to learn fully,

the pace is deliberate and most people find the practice
deeply satisfying.

To find a class, contact the Tai Chi Union for Great Britain
(www.taichiunion.com), which is a collective of more than
500 independent instructors around the country.

244 **Pilates** – This ultra-fashionable technique was
once the preserve of dancers, actors, film stars
and sportspeople, but is now more widely available to all of
us. Instead of focusing on how much exercise we do, Pilates –
which bears the name of the German boxer, circus performer
and self-defence teacher who created it in the early-twentieth
century – emphasises quality. With a slow pace, paying
attention to the alignment of your body and exploring what
a particular exercise feels like, the idea is that you start
'thinking in activity' rather than just 'getting it done'.

The aim of Pilates is not to develop those muscles in the body
that are already powerful, but to strengthen the weaker ones
– particularly those concerned with posture and what Pilates
called the 'girdle of strength', meaning our back, belly and
bum. The result is a long, lean physique with a firm 'core'.

Most people begin Pilates with a matwork class, using small
pieces of equipment and their own body weight to add
resistance during calm and very focused routines. Once you've

grasped the principles, you might move on to use some of the machines – such as the universal reformer, a sliding bed with springs attached – which Pilates devised and which has hardly changed in three-quarters of a century.

While matwork is taught in small groups of up to ten people, you might receive personal tuition on the machines or work with a couple of others receiving slightly less guidance. That's why machine classes are more expensive than matwork, but you'll quickly notice the difference if you find a good instructor. You'll finish a session feeling eight feet tall and beautifully toned.

There are now plenty of books and DVDs you can use at home to continue the good work, or your teacher will give you a set of exercises to practise between classes.

To find a teacher, contact the Pilates Foundation UK (www.pilatesfouundation.com) or Body Control Pilates (www.bodycontrol.co.uk).

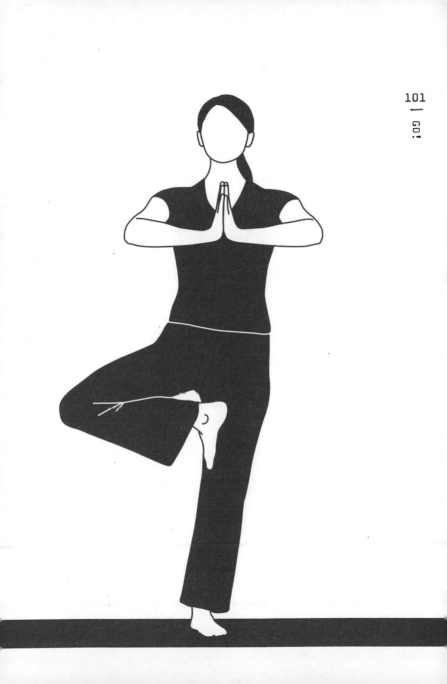

MY TOP TIPS

FIND A TRAINING BUDDY

'FIND SOMEONE WITH THE SAME ASPIRATIONS AS YOU. SET A DATE AND TIME SO YOU CAN'T BACK OUT. IT'S CHEAPER THAN A PERSONAL TRAINER!'

GET OFF THE BUS EARLY

'IF IT'S A NICE DAY WALK THE LAST MILE. WALKING IS THE EASIEST WAY TO BUILD ACTIVITY INTO YOUR DAY.'

DITCH THE CHOCOLATE
'DON'T GRAB A
CHOCOLATE BAR AT
LUNCHTIME BECAUSE
YOU'RE STILL HUNGRY;
GET USED TO HEALTHY
GRAZING THROUGH THE
DAY. RAISINS MIGHT
NOT BE YOUR THING BUT
PLENTY OF FRUIT IS NOW
PACKAGED FOR SNACKING.'

DENISE LEWIS
OLYMPIC HEPTATHLON GOLD
MEDALLIST

WORK WORK WORKOUT!

Activity in the office shouldn't just be limited to clicking your mouse and picking up the phone.

245 **Don't send an email to a colleague** somewhere else in the building – walk to her desk and talk to her instead. As well as being good exercise, it's also very sociable! Why not see if your organisation will institute some office games to get the workforce more active? Whether it's lunchtime walking groups or 'email-free Fridays', there are plenty of ideas to help everyone move around more.

246 **Don't make internal phone calls,** for the same reason.

247 **Open envelopes with your fingers** rather than a letter opener. This keeps your finger and thumb muscles active, possibly preventing arthritis.

248 **Lift the bin up with your feet** before putting litter in. This works your thigh and lower abdominal muscles.

249 **Be the office gopher.** No matter what your status, make regular trips to the kitchen to prepare drinks for everyone.

250 **If your chair has casters, use it to move around the office.** Sitting upright and pulling it with the balls of the feet is a great hamstring toner.

251 **Don't keep a bottle of water on your desk –** keep walking back and forth to the cooler. Each minute spent doing so burns six calories.

252 **Changing the water container works the chest** when the bottle is hugged, the thighs and lower back when it's picked up, and the abs throughout.

253 **Keep a pair of training shoes, some workout kit and a towel underneath your desk** or in your locker. It's harder to make excuses when everything you need to exercise is there waiting for you.

254 **Almost every workplace has stairs** – so use them instead of the lift. If you're on the 101st floor, then you're excused walking up the lot – but why not get out at the 98th and finish your journey on foot? Climbing 3,407m (10,200ft) of stairs is the equivalent of completing the Three Peaks Challenge! (By the way, if you do actually fancy climbing the highest mountains in England, Scotland and Wales within 24 hours, check out the website www.3peaks.info for full details.)

255 **Don't be shy about telling your colleagues that you are trying to build more activity into your everyday life.** Not only might they want to join you and forsake the after-work trip to the pub in favour of a game of badminton or run in the park, your employer may be inspired to offer a discounted gym or sports club membership, or set up weekly yoga and Pilates sessions in the boardroom.

256 **Organise your workstation** so that items you use regularly are not always within easy reach. That way, you'll have to stand up and stretch more often.

257 **If you travel to work by public transport,** start and finish your journey a stop early to add an invigorating walk in the morning and a more relaxing stroll as you wind down later in the day.

258 **On the phone a lot?** Don't slouch in your seat, feet on your desk, receiver crushed between shoulder and ear: stand up while you're speaking and, if you have a cordless phone, move around. As well as giving your muscles some gentle work to do, many people find this approach also helps them to speak more fluently and confidently.

259 **Too busy for exercise?** The key is to make time work for you. Coffee break? Lunchtime mooch around the shops munching a sandwich? Afternoon tea and chat break? Add them together and an hour will magically appear which you can put to much better use. Even a short 20-minute walk can make a difference. Your productivity will probably increase, too.

260 **So where exactly does the woman in the next office go every lunchtime** before returning 45 minutes later with damp hair and rosy cheeks? Don't be afraid to ask – she'll probably offer to take you along as well.

261 **Set yourself an office challenge.** How about climbing Mount Everest (without the snow)? Or walking from the Angel of the North to the Tower of London without having to leave the building? You'll find everything you need to set up such challenges at www.sportengland.org/getactive.

BEST FOOT FORWARD

Think of running as a faster version of walking. Just as we pay attention to the sound of our feet on the ground, the smoothness of our stride, our posture and economy of movement when we walk, so we can do exactly the same when we pick up the pace a little. By doing this, running becomes an activity where the process (what it feels like to run) matters more than the end result (how far or how fast). This is the key to keeping going.

262 **If you're new to running, don't set yourself targets.** Your first few runs should be nothing more than a process of discovery: can I run from my house to the trees across the park? And if I can, what about running back again? Is this a comfortable pace? Does it feel easy – or will I have to stop after a couple of hundred paces?

263 **Remember, you're not in training for a marathon** – that might come later! You're simply exploring an activity that, for a 70kg (154 lb) man, can burn a massive 550 calories per hour even at a very comfortable 8kph (5mph).

'MOVE EVERY DAY. THAT HAS TO BE YOUR FOUNDATION. DON'T BEAT YOURSELF UP IF YOU DON'T GET TO THE GYM, DO THINGS YOU ENJOY. AND GET OUT AND WALK! IT'S THE CHEAPEST AND MOST ACCESSIBLE BODY-SHAPING ACTIVITY OF ALL.'

JOANNA HALL

FITNESS EXPERT, WRITER AND TV PRESENTER

264 **On your first few outings, you may find yourself walking as much as running.** This is fine. Begin by walking for two minutes, then jogging for 30 seconds, then walking for two minutes, and so on. Try to make smooth transitions between each phase so you're not jerking your body along, and think about 'running tall' so you lift your torso up out of your hips.

265 **Try not to land heavily on your heels,** but find a position where your body is upright and the weight when you land is more towards the front of your feet, with your feet directly underneath your body rather than shooting out in front of you. Look forward rather than down at the ground, so your head is nicely balanced on your neck and spine.

266 **As your fitness improves, you can vary the time spent walking and running,** until you reach your first achievement: being able to run for longer than you walk. Gradually reduce the walking intervals until you are able to run at a steady pace – not so fast that you would be unable to chat to a friend – for ten minutes.

267 **Joining a local running group is a great way to keep putting one foot in front of the other.** There's no need to worry that everyone will be ultra-speedy and will leave you trailing in their wake – most groups split up into fast, medium, slow and super-slow, with someone on hand to look after you. Many groups are based at a local sports centre, so ask there or pop into your nearest sports shop to get information. Alternatively, browse the databases at www.runtrackdir.com/ukclubs or http://running.timeoutdoors.com/clubs.

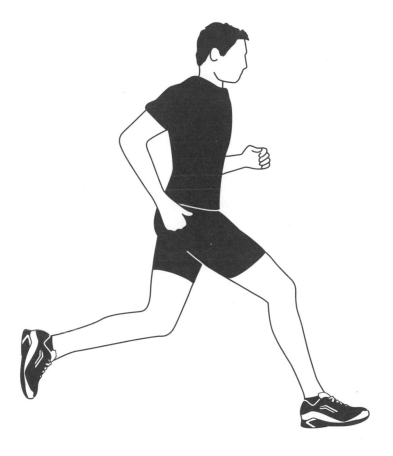

268 The Sisters Network can put you in touch with other women in your area who want to run or jog together. There are groups all round the country who meet at regular times. For details, visit www.croydon-running-sisters.org.uk/sisnet.

269 There are lots of organised runs you can enter to set yourself a challenge. It doesn't have to be the London Marathon – why not start with a small, local fun run over three miles or five kilometres, and get a friend to sign up with you? You can find hundreds of runs listed at www.runnersworld.co.uk/events.

270 The Race for Life women-only 5k runs raise funds for breast cancer research, and there are more than 230 events around the country to choose from. Contact www.raceforlife.org to find out more.

THE NUMBERS GAME

271

Over-indulged on the chocolate?

There are 684 calories in a third of a box of
Mars Celebrations.

Don't worry!

For a 70kg (154lb) man to burn them off and give
the heart and lungs a workout, he can do:

Two hours of easy cycling.

90 minutes of brisk hill walking.

Or a 40-minute run at 14kph (9mph).

TAKE THE PLUNGE

There's one big reason why it's vital for everyone to swim competently: one day, it may save your life or someone else's. So if you can't swim at all or feel you need to improve your confidence in the water, why not book a course of lessons? Qualified instructors are sympathetic to any issues you may have, such as putting your face under the surface. Ask for details at your local pool.

272 **Swimming is great all-round exercise,** building stamina, strength and suppleness. It uses every major muscle group, so it will tone and shape your body.

273 **As it is an aerobic activity,** swimming will keep your heart and lungs healthy and can help you lose weight.

274 **Swimming is a low-impact sport,** so there's no weight-bearing involved. That makes it ideal for anyone with back problems or arthritis, for women who are pregnant, or for people with disabilities.

275 **Splashing around in a pool is a fantastic energiser.** A lunchtime swim will prevent an afternoon slump.

276 **This form of exercise is good for asthmatics.** The humid air around a swimming pool makes breathing more comfortable.

277 **At first, don't worry about how far or how fast you swim.** Simply enjoy the feeling of being in the water. Vary your strokes so that you exercise different muscle groups, and really work on your technique.

278 **Too many people swim with their head out of the water,** placing strain on the neck and spine and preventing them using their whole body more efficiently. Think streamlined! Wearing goggles makes it easier to swim for long periods with your face submerged.

279 **Gradually build up the number of lengths you can swim in a 30-minute session,** or the number you can complete without stopping for a breather. By completing one length in 30 seconds and swimming steadily for half an hour, a 57kg (126lb) woman will burn a fantastic 210 calories.

280 **Race other people in the pool,** whether they know what you're doing or not.

281 **Time your lengths** and try to improve your times or distances with each visit.

282 **Don't just swim:** use the resistance of the water for powerwalking or running.

283 **Play throwing and catching games** if you're allowed, or if the pool is empty.

284 **Rubber rings and floats** are not only for non-swimmers – use them to help you vary your workout.

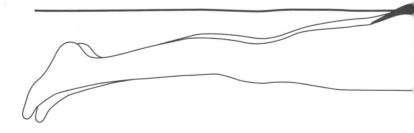

285 **When taking children to a lido,** don't just sit in the sun or at the bar while the kids play. Join in with their fun.

286 **If relaxing in the sauna,** don't just flop out. Heat makes your muscles, joints and ligaments more flexible, so do some stretching exercises.

287 **When sitting in a whirlpool spa,** use the jets of water as resistance against which to press your arms, legs and back.

288 **Even in a fun pool, you can enhance your swimming workout.** Swim against the tide in the 'lazy river' and ride the waves when the wave machine is turned on.

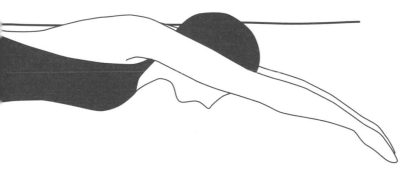

289 **As you throw a diving toy into the pool,** state a 5- or 10-point value. Whoever retrieves the toy wins the points. The first to 50 is the champion diver.

290 **When you're taking a break from swimming lengths,** hold on to the end of the pool, bring your knees together and twist your legs from side to side – a good flexibility exercise for the back and abdominal muscles.

291 **Since it began in 1986, more than half a million people have taken part in the Swimathon,** and swum 900,000km (570,000 miles) to raise funds for charity – that's 23 times around the earth! This annual event sets a range of challenges that are achievable by everyone, either on your own or as part of a team. You don't even have to swim the distance in one go – you can log your laps over several days. For details of the next Swimathon click on www.swimathon.org.

'PHYSICAL FITNESS IS
NOT ONLY ONE OF THE
MOST IMPORTANT KEYS
TO A HEALTHY BODY,
IT IS THE BASIS OF
DYNAMIC AND CREATIVE
INTELLECTUAL ACTIVITY.
INTELLIGENCE AND SKILL
CAN ONLY FUNCTION AT
THE PEAK OF THEIR
CAPACITY WHEN THE
BODY IS HEALTHY AND
STRONG.'

JOHN F. KENNEDY
AMERICAN PRESIDENT

ON YOUR BIKE

Cycling has wheel appeal – and green appeal, too. Three-quarters of the journeys we make are 8km (5 miles) or less, costing us money in terms of the petrol our cars guzzle and damaging the environment every time we turn on the engine. Most of those journeys could be covered on a bike – and, in many towns and cities, more quickly as well.

A study carried out for the Department of Transport found that even a small amount of cycling can have a real impact on fitness levels. The study showed that aerobic fitness increased by 11 per cent after just six weeks of cycling short distances, four times a week. If people cycled 6km (4 miles) to and from work, in total, each day, the aerobic benefit would increase to 17 per cent. People who don't exercise at all, but who start cycling, can move from the third of the population who are the least fit to being among the fittest in just a few months.

Need any more convincing that getting on your bike is a great idea?

292 **You can whizz past those drivers stuck in a queue.** On reasonably flat ground, you can cover 6km (4 miles) in half an hour.

293 **Cycling can help you lose weight.** An hour of steady riding burns about 300 calories – the amount in a Mars bar or a pint and a half of beer. A 15-minute ride to and from work, five times a week, will burn the equivalent of 5kg (11lb) of fat in a year!

294 **Cyclists and pedestrians actually absorb lower levels of pollutants than car drivers,** so if you're concerned about the potential damage caused by traffic fumes, don't be.

295 **Cycling is good aerobic exercise,** reducing the risk of conditions such as heart disease, high blood pressure, obesity and diabetes, and can help to maintain strength and coordination.

296 **Just as importantly, cycling is good fun!** And because it's fun, it can reduce stress levels, boost self-esteem and put us in a good mood.

297 **Cycling is for everyone,** whether on your own, with a partner or as a family. If you're new to it, begin by using your bike to pop down the road to the shops or the postbox, then gradually increase the distance and frequency. A basket or pannier will enable you to carry items such as shopping.

298 **Why not plan a family outing by bike?** It could be a simple ride to a local park, or you could journey further afield. You can take your bike on many trains (check with the operator before setting out) and on the overground sections of the London Underground outside peak hours. Pack a picnic and a map and make a day of it.

299 **Don't cycle in a single gears.** Change up and down to vary your workout.

300 **When cycling up a steep hill, don't get off and push.** Use the gears to help you with the ascent, and feel a real sense of achievement at the top.

301 **Time regular journeys,** and begin leaving the house slightly later on each occasion while still aiming to arrive on time.

302 **On a weekend ride, lower the saddle slightly.** This will force you to stand up more often to pedal, offering a tougher workout.

303 **Devise a 'treasure hunt'.** Everyone has to suggest two or three objects to find during a bike ride. The first person to complete the list is the winner (prize optional).

Whether you're riding on busy roads or quiet country lanes, you must wear a correctly fitting helmet. Seek expert advice from a bike shop. Other than a repair kit for those occasional punctures, you don't need any further specialist equipment.

304 British Cycling (www.everydaycycling.com) is a great source of information on cycle routes and trails, charity rides and various two-wheel sports including BMX, road and track cycling and mountain-biking.

305 Why not set yourself the challenge of taking part in one of the major sponsored bike rides that are held around the country each summer? The London to Brighton Ride is the best known and most popular, but others include the Oxford to Cambridge, the Norwich Bike Ride, the Portsmouth and Langstone 'Round the Harbours', and the London to Paris Team Relay. You'll certainly find something in your area, over a distance that's achievable.

Not only are they fun to enter, either on your own, with a partner or friends, or as a family, but having a target to aim for will keep you motivated while you exercise. And if you raise sponsorship, you'll be helping other people, too.

306

The British Heart Foundation organises many of the major sponsored rides, along with other events such as walks, runs, swims and parachute jumps, as part of its Hearts First Challenge series. To find out more visit www.bhf.org.uk/events.

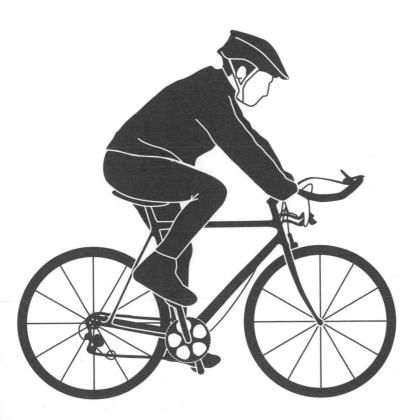

POSTURE PERFECT

Ask a friend to stand up straight. The chances are she will pull back her shoulders and puff out her chest, like a sergeant major. By doing this, she is in fact stiffening her body. When it comes to moving, someone who stands like this will look strangely robotic.

307 **Good posture doesn't mean forcing your body into a fixed position.** It means being aware of how you are sitting, standing, walking, swimming or running – and thinking about how you can eliminate any tension that might be building up as a result. Good posture will help your body to function more efficiently, and will make you look taller and slimmer. It also improves blood circulation, keeps energy levels up and reduces the risk of back pain caused by persistent slouching or excessive curvature of the spine.

Stand up and look at your feet. Are they pointing slightly outwards, at 11 o'clock and 1 o'clock, which is a comfortable position for most of us? Or are they turned further out towards 10 o'clock and 2 o'clock? Or is one pointing in a completely different direction to the other?

- When you're standing at ease, do you place your weight on one hip (bad), or stand straight with your weight equally distributed (good)?
- Are your shoulders up around your neck (bad) or relaxed and down (good)?
- Is your spine lengthened and relaxed (good), or is your pelvis thrust forward (bad)?
- Is your head balanced on your spine (good), or can you feel tension at the back of your neck (bad)?
- If you lean forward, do you lean from your hips (good) or by curving your shoulders and upper back (bad)?
- When you pick something off the ground, do you bend your knees (good) or your back (bad)?

With practice, we can all improve our posture and learn to move effortlessly and gracefully.

AT A STRETCH

Everyone loses around 2cm (¾in) in height between getting up in the morning and going to bed at night. This is caused by the compression of spinal discs during daytime activities. All the more reason, then, to stand tall and s-t-r-e-t-c-h!

308 **When you get up, take a few seconds to stand tall, breathe in and raise your fingers to the sky.** Feel your spine extending.

309 **Use stairs and steps for stretching and strengthening.** With the balls of your feet on the edge of a step, slowly lower your heels until you feel a stretch in your calf muscles. Now rise up until you can feel your calf muscles contract. This is a good exercise for oft-neglected muscles.

310 **Hang loose!** An outdoor fire escape is the perfect place from which to hang with your arms fully extended. Your shoulders will get a great stretch, and your spine will lengthen and straighten – countering the compression forced upon it by everyday sitting and standing.

311 **If you spend much of the day sitting at a computer, take regular screen breaks.** Lean back in your chair, clasp your hands behind your head and feel a stretch across your shoulders. Now lean forward and drop your head between your knees to stretch your lower back. Clasp your hands behind your back and pull your elbows towards each other to stretch across the front of your chest. Now stretch your arms out in front of you and clasp your hands. Tuck your chin into your chest to feel a stretch through your upper back.

312 **In the evening, lie on the floor and lift your feet up with your knees together.** Clasp your hands behind your knees, then lift your head and shoulders to feel a stretch in the lower back.

313 **Finally, rest on hands and knees with a flat back,** then arch your back upwards to feel a stretch through the length of the spine.

CHILL OUT

Whenever you've been out for a walk, a run or digging the garden, take ten minutes afterwards for what is called 'active rest'.

314 Lie on a firm surface with your head supported by a rolled-up towel or a paperback book, with your legs bent and knees pointing to the sky. Allow your hands to rest comfortably by your side, elbows pointing outwards. Keep your eyes open.

This is a great way to:
- Release tension.
- Reconnect with your body.
- Practise breathing deeply and steadily.
- Regain your length (the average person loses around 2cm (¾in) in height between waking up in the morning and going to bed at night.)
- Think about the activity you've just done – the progress you've made and how much you're looking forward to doing it again next time.

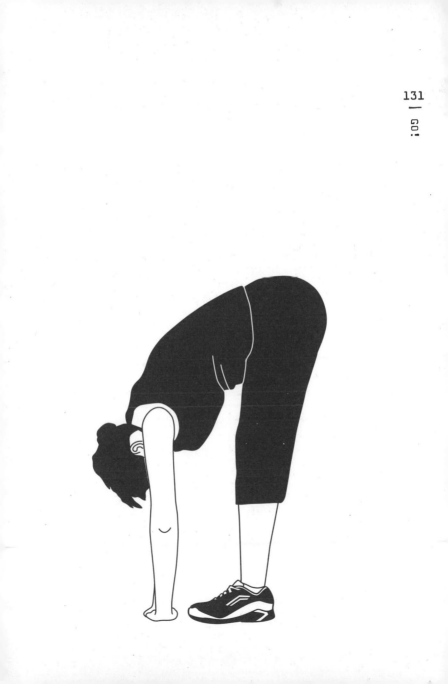

VOLUNTEER

Every organisation welcomes helpers, whether you've got plenty of free time or can only devote the occasional hour here and there. Volunteering is also a great way to make new friends and to get active, particularly outdoors. For more information go to www.volunteering.org.

315 **Why not learn a new skill, such as stone-walling or ditch digging,** from the British Trust for Conservation Volunteers (www.btcv.org.uk)? There are groups all over Britain helping to care for landscapes both rural and urban. You can burn a third more calories in an hour of some Green Gym activities than in a step aerobics class, while lifting, carrying, digging, pulling and building are great for strength, flexibility and toning. Plus there's the satisfaction of a good job done.

316 **Many parks have a management group** drawn from local residents who help build paths, clear copses and keep trees and hedges in trim. Ask at your local council office.

317 **Too old to play football?** You're never too old to become a referee and enjoy a good run-out on Saturday afternoons. Training courses are arranged locally: contact the Football Association (www.theFA.com).

318 **Sports clubs always need helpers.** If you're a keen gardener you could help with the upkeep of the ground; DIY fans could keep the clubhouse looking smart. Or you could simply offer to put out the flags around the pitch on match days.

319 **If there's a sport you particularly enjoy or used to play,** why not learn to become a coach and volunteer at a local club? All sports have an introductory qualification: the course will teach you the basics of coaching and allow you to assist more experienced coaches. Sport England (www.sportengland.org/getactive) will point you in the right direction.

320 **Is there a local club for people with physical disabilities?** Pushing a wheelchair is both helpful and great all-round exercise!

A SIMPLE GUIDE TO EATING WELL

A calorie is a measure of the energy value of food. On average, men need to consume around 2,500 calories per day to maintain their body weight, women around 2,000. However, this depends on how much energy you expend and the fuel you take on board.

If you consume 2,000 calories in a typical day and also expend 2,000, your calorific balance is neutral and your weight will not change.

If you consume 2,500 calories in a typical day and expend 2,000, your calorific balance is negative and you will put on weight.

One way of trying to lose weight is by reducing your calorie intake. So if you now consume 1,600 calories in a typical day but still expend 2,000, your calorific balance is positive and you will lose weight.

Regular activity helps to speed up your metabolic rate – that is, the rate at which your body naturally burns up calories.

Since food is a pleasure to be enjoyed, this last option is the best way to stay healthy, lose weight and improve your shape: eat the same amount of food but do more exercise.

An excellent introduction to healthy eating and good nutrition can be found at the British Nutrition Foundation's website: www.nutrition.org.uk.

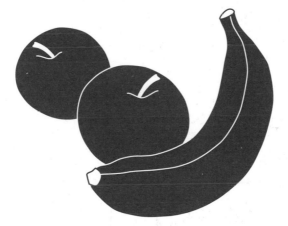

Generally speaking, no one food type is bad: it's how much of it we eat that is the key issue. We often hear talk of a 'balanced diet'. What exactly does that mean?

321 **Carbohydrates:** These are our main source of energy, and around 55–60 per cent of our daily calorie intake should come from 'carbs'. Try to gain as much as possible from complex carbohydrates such as cereals, bread, pulses and rice, which release their energy slowly and bring other nutrients, rather than from simple carbohydrates such as chocolate, biscuits, cakes and sugary drinks, which only give an instant 'hit' of energy and offer few other nutritional benefits. Excess carbohydrate is stored by the body as fat.

322 **Protein:** This is used by the body to build and repair muscles and tissues, and should provide around 15–20 per cent of daily calorie intake. Good sources of protein can come from vegetable products as well as animal ones: meat, fish, nuts, milk, eggs, cheese and pulses such as lentils and chickpeas.

323 **Fats:** Despite its image, fat is just as important as the other nutrients in food. The problem is that most of us eat too much of it, and don't differentiate between saturated and unsaturated fats. In total, no more than 25 per cent of our daily calorie intake should come from fats.

A small amount of saturated fat is not harmful, but too much of it can raise blood cholesterol levels, which also increases the risk of heart disease. Most saturated fat comes from animal-based foods such as dairy products, meat, lard, cakes, biscuits and snack products. Some vegetable-based foods, including coconut, palm oil and cocoa butter, are also high in saturated fat.

Unsaturated fats mainly come from plant sources and can be further divided into monounsaturates and polyunsaturates according to their chemical composition. These types of fats are a good source of essential fatty acids. Foods high in monounsaturated fat include avocados, cashews, olives and peanuts, plus olive and peanut oils. Foods high in polyunsaturated fat include soft margarine, mayonnaise, salad dressing, most nuts and some seeds, plus corn, sesame and soybean oils.

Some fish contain a type of polyunsaturated fat called omega-3 fatty acids. These are termed essential fatty acids because the body cannot make them, and they must be obtained from our food. That's why oily fish such as mackerel, herring, salmon and trout are such healthy options.

324

Fibre: Eating lots of fruit, vegetables and grains will ensure that your diet is rich in fibre – the bulk that not only helps us to feel full but also moves food through the digestive system and 'keeps us regular'. Fibre-rich foods are usually low in calories and crammed with protein, complex carbohydrates, vitamins and minerals. Fibre also lowers cholesterol levels, stabilises blood sugar and has a major part to play in preventing conditions such as bowel cancer. Aim to eat 20g (¾oz) of fibre daily: you can work out how much you're consuming from the nutritional information provided on food packaging.

325

Vitamins and minerals: We only need these substances in small quantities but their impact on the body is huge. Like oil in a car engine, they keep everything moving smoothly – and we really notice the effects of a deficiency. Dull hair, dry skin, bruises and cuts that take ages to heal, brittle nails – these are all signs that we may lack certain vitamins and minerals. A multi-vitamin and mineral supplement is one way to ensure a balance, but a far better approach is through good nutrition. A balanced and varied diet which includes plenty of fresh fruit and vegetables will do the trick without the need for a trip to the pharmacist.

326 **Water:** We can survive without food for relatively long periods, but we can't survive without water. It comprises about 75–80 per cent of our body weight and is vital for transporting good chemicals around the body, absorbing the nutrients from food, dissolving the waste from food and regulating body temperature. You will need to drink more if you are exercising. However, few of us drink anything like enough water – far too much of our fluid intake comes from tea, coffee, fizzy drinks and alcohol. You should never reach the point where you are thirsty: aim to drink at least 1.5 litres (2.5 pints) of still water each day. It doesn't matter matter whether it's from a bottle or the tap. If you're planning a long drive, keep a bottle (with an easy-to-remove lid) to hand in the car.

327 **Pop a bottle in your bag before setting out to work,** and sip it throughout your journey.

328 **Most offices have a watercooler:** every time you pass it, pour yourself a cup.

329 Pack a bottle in a lunchbox in preference to a carton of sugary drink.

330 If you can't do without some flavouring, mix water 50–50 with fruit juice or add a small amount of fruit squash.

You might need to visit the loo slightly more often, but think of it as internal cleansing!

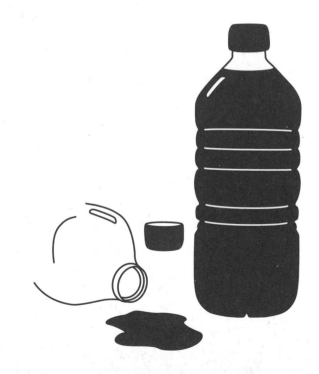

331 **Exercise is likely to make you feel hungry.** It's important to use this as an opportunity to refuel with foods that are nutritious and naturally low in calories rather than crammed with fat, sugar and salt. Grazing on small amounts of food at regular intervals throughout the day will stop your tummy rumbling and prevent the energy dip that affects many people in mid-afternoon and which often sends them to the biscuit tin or to buy a bar of chocolate.

Dried or fresh fruit, unsalted nuts, malt loaf, sticks of raw vegetables (perhaps with a low-fat dip), rice cakes and wholegrain crackers will all stave off hunger pangs without adding hundreds of empty calories to your daily intake.

Some foods have got the lot – they are nutritious, tasty and able to prevent or fight off all kinds of illnesses. Try and incorporate these top ten in your diet:

332 **Avocado:** Packed with vitamins, potassium and monounsaturated fats.

333 **Beans:** Fresh or dried, they're high in protein, fibre and iron and low in fat.

334 **Blueberries:** A great source of vitamin C, folic acid, fibre and hundreds of other compounds. Blueberries also have a very thick skin, which is where nature packs most of its nutrients.

335 **Broccoli:** Like other cruciferous vegetables such as cauliflower, kale, Brussels sprouts and cabbage, broccoli is rich in iron, beta-carotene and vitamin C.

336 **Carrots:** You can get your entire daily intake of vitamin A from a single carrot, not to mention calcium, iron, potassium and vitamins B and C.

337 **Garlic:** Renowned for lowering the risk of heart disease and stroke, boosting circulation, reducing cholesterol, and protecting against colds, coughs and flu.

338 **Oats:** A food with a slow energy release, which can cut cholesterol levels and is rich in vitamins B and E plus many minerals.

339 **Peppers:** Red and yellow peppers in particular are high in vitamin C, beta-carotene, iron and potassium.

340 **Sprouted seeds:** A powerhouse store of vitamins, minerals and enzymes. The seeds actually become more nutritious as they grow. What's more, you can sprout your own in a glass jar or plastic sprouter in 3–5 days – for the cost of just a few pence.

341 **Watercress:** Rich in vitamins A, B and C, potassium, zinc and other minerals, watercress also helps to prevent anaemia and eczema and protects against more serious diseases.

GLYCAEMIC INDEX

342 **The glycaemic index** – currently fashionable as the GI diet – measures the effect on blood sugar levels of eating particular foods (compared to pure glucose, which is rated 100 on the index). Foods with a low GI rating (below 50) are absorbed by the body more slowly than those with a high GI (above 70), thus affecting blood sugar levels less dramatically and giving a steady release of energy. Try to eat plenty of low GI foods to balance out energy peaks and troughs through the day. A comprehensive guide to the GI ratings of different foods can be found at www.glycaemicindex.com. Here's a selection:

Apples	30
Apple juice (fresh)	40
Bananas	65
Broccoli	10
Chocolate	70
Cornflakes	85
Grapes	40
Green vegetables	10
Honey	90
Jam	65
Milk (semi-skimmed)	30
Oranges	35
Peanuts	20
Popcorn (no sugar)	85
Potatoes (peeled and boiled)	70
Potato crisps	80
Pumpkin	75
Raisins	65
Rice (basmati)	50
Rice (pre-cooked)	90
Tomatoes	10
Walnuts	15
White pasta	55
Yoghurt (whole milk)	35

343 We should aim to eat five varied portions of fruit and vegetables a day as a minimum.

One portion of fruit is, for example, half a large grapefruit, a slice of melon or two satsumas. Dried fruit also counts – for example, one portion would be three dried apricots, or a tablespoon of raisins. A glass of 100 per cent fruit or vegetable juice counts as one portion – but you can only count juice as one portion per day, no matter how much you drink. This is because it has very little fibre.

One portion of vegetables is, for example, three tablespoonfuls of cooked carrots or peas or sweetcorn, or a cereal bowl of mixed salad. Beans and other pulses such as kidney beans, lentils and chick peas count only once a day, no matter how much you eat. While pulses contain fibre, they don't contain the same mixture of vitamins, minerals and other nutrients as fruit and vegetables. Potatoes don't count towards your five a day because they are a starchy food.

For more information, visit www.5aday.nhs.uk.

Once eating five portions a day becomes part of your life, why stop? Try and build up to ten!

344 **Eat raw food every day:** precious minerals, vitamins and enzymes can be damaged or lost during cooking, so eat raw fruit and vegetables whenever possible!

345 **When you do need to cook veg, steam rather than boil.** That way, the valuable nutrients stay in the food rather than disappear into the water.

346 **Frozen fruit and veg are not only convenient, they're often fresher than fresh goods!** Peas, for example, go from pod to packet in just a few hours.

347 **Look at the colours on your plate:** if there's an attractive mix of hues, it's a fair bet the meal you've prepared is balanced and nutritious.

348 **Herbs are not only nutritious and therapeutic,** they're easily and cheaply grown for a few pence on a sunny windowsill. Why pay for a supermarket bunch of parsley or mint when you can pick leaves fresh from a plant?

349 When buying food, remember these simple guidelines: in 100g (3½oz) of a product, 2g of sugars is a little but 10g is a lot; 3g of total fat is a little but 20g is a lot; 1g of saturated fat is a little but 5g is a lot.

350 Reduce the amount of fat you use by grilling food instead of frying. If you have to fry, use a spray oil (instead of a pouring oil or a solid fat like lard, margarine or butter).

351 Bread or potatoes are not fattening, but the spread or oil you put on them bumps up the calories. Either cut back on butter and margarine or choose low-fat alternatives.

352 Eating healthily doesn't have to be expensive. Instead of buying all your fruit and veg on a single weekly shop, buy smaller amounts more often if you have time. Not only will this be more economical, it means the produce will be fresher.

353 There's absolutely nothing wrong with having a bar of chocolate, a beer, a burger or a takeaway. Just remember two watchwords: balance and moderation.

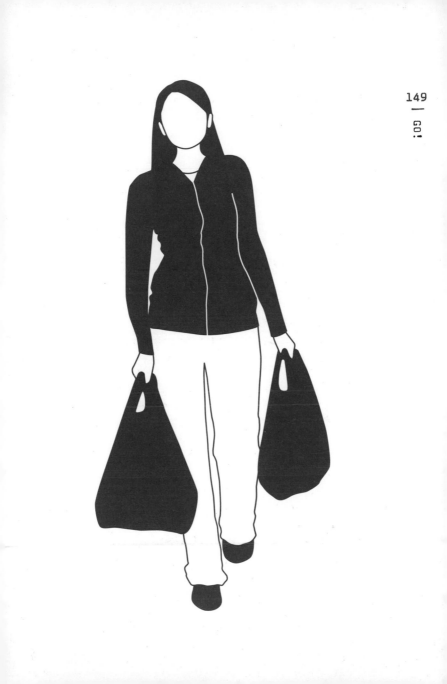

KEEPING IT UP

354 **Variety is the spice of life** – and exercise, too. Don't try just one sport or fitness activity, try lots!

355 **Don't worry about not knowing the rules or being one step behind the rest of the class.** Remember, everyone was a beginner once.

356 **If you don't like the gym, don't go!** Do something else you enjoy instead.

357 **Make a commitment.** Write down what you plan to do in your diary amd arrange other things around your exercise sessions.

358 **Decide which days and times are best for you to exercise and stick to them.**

359 **Don't choose an activity because you think it might be good for you.** The first question you should always ask is: will I enjoy it?

360 **Don't give up if you have a bad week.** It happens to us all.

361 **Find someone to exercise with.** Getting fit doesn't have to be a solitary pursuit.

362 **Not everyone finds exercise immediately enjoyable.** Some of us have bad memories from schooldays, or are stuck with the idea that it has to be painful or spartan. But stick with it – your opinion may change once you start to look and feel fitter and healthier.

363 **Don't push yourself too hard,** especially at first. Enthusiasm is good, pain is not – it's a sign that something is wrong.

364 **Try to do something that raises your heart rate every day of the week.**

365 **Smile!** Even when you're tired or it's tough, keep smiling!

FITNESS FACTS

HOW OFTEN SHOULD I EXERCISE?

Over the years, there have been lots of different theories about how much exercise we need to do in order to stay fit. You might have heard some fitness experts say: 'At least three times a week, at moderate to high intensity, for a minimum of 30 minutes.'

That's a useful ideal. However, the good news is that any exercise, whatever its duration and intensity, can help. That's why it's so vital to build as much activity as possible into our everyday lives, rather than making a commitment to go to the gym that, a few weeks later, looks unappealing and impractical.

What's remarkable is that someone who walks to work every day, who climbs the office stairs instead of using the lift, who enjoys physical play with his or her children and who is a keen gardener may actually possess more 'functional fitness' than a three-times-a-week gym slave!

ALL IN THE GENES?

Some of the factors affecting fitness are hereditary and we can't do much about them. Others, however, are firmly within our sphere of influence.

Let's start with the hereditary ones first.

BODY TYPE

There are three basic body types: skinny, athletic and rounded. We can't change our type but physical activity and sensible eating will improve our shape and help us to make the most of our particular type.

The scientific term for a skinny body type is ectomorphic. An ectomorph is long and lean, with narrow shoulders and hips, a small bone structure and a low level of body fat. Most endurance athletes are ectomorphs – think of Paula Radcliffe and you'll get the picture. Ectomorphs find it easy to lose weight and keep it off, and often excel at cardiovascular activities such as long-distance running. However, they can appear fragile and prone to injury.

An athletic body type is known as mesomorphic. A mesomorph is broad shouldered with a narrow waist and a powerful look. Gymnasts, sprinters, rugby players and rowers are good examples of mesomorphs. However, they can put on weight quickly if they stop exercising and lose all the benefits of their earlier activity.

The term for the rounded body type is endomorphic. Endomorphs are usually short, with a wide frame and not much muscle definition. They gain weight easily and can carry too much body fat – but are often strong and good at activities requiring power.

Very few people fit perfectly into one of these three types. Most of us are mainly one type with a bit of another. It's important to remember that no one body type is superior to another – all three have advantages and disadvantages when it comes to being active and developing fitness. And it's very easy for a beer-drinking, burger-munching mesomorph to look more like an endomorph than someone of that build who exercises regularly and eats well.

GENDER

At one time it was usually men who went out and played sport. Today, many women take part in sport, although they are more likely to face obstacles such as lack of time and money and the need for childcare. For some, there are also cultural sensitivities and issues of self-esteem.

This book makes no distinctions. All the ideas featured here are suitable for both men and women. However, an increasing number of sports centres, clubs and groups offer women-only sessions for those who prefer single-sex activities.

AGE

'Oh, I'm too old to…' What exactly?

No one is too old to do anything. Age is not a barrier to exercise, and there are countless inspiring stories of 90-year-old marathon runners and swimmers to back that belief. Of course, we may not all want to indulge in such dramatic feats but, as we get older, one thing is indisputably true: inactivity leads to an inability to be active. Unused muscles grow weak, joints stiffen and a body that still has so much potential is left to decline.

By the way, the women's over-70s world long jump record is well in excess of 4m (13 ft). Get a tape and measure it out! Inspiring?

Now, let's turn to two major factors that we have the power to change: smoking and nutrition.

SMOKING

Smoking doubles the risk of premature death from heart disease. Someone who smokes 40 a day is 20 times more likely to die of lung cancer than a non-smoker.

Factor in numerous other gruesome cancers, gum disease, lower sperm counts for men, potential damage to an unborn baby for pregnant women, kidney disease, smoker's cough and bronchial infections, and it's clear why smoking is the number one health hazard and preventable cause of death.

A smoker has a faster heart rate and uses oxygen less efficiently than a non-smoker – but if you quit and start to exercise, your body will begin to heal itself. If you can stay off the fags for ten years, you'll undo most of the damage.

NUTRITION

Poor eating habits leave us lacking energy and at risk of conditions such as diabetes, heart disease and osteoporosis – not to mention the epidemic of obesity afflicting the Western world.

We are what we eat – and if we are to become more active, increased physical activity will make extra demands on the body. If we don't replenish our energy with the right foods and a balance of protein, carbohydrates, fat, fibre, minerals and vitamins, we run the risk of becoming run down and undoing all the good work of exercising.

'A Simple Guide to Eating Well' earlier in this book will get you started.

MYTHS - AND HITS!

WEIGHT TRAINING TURNS WOMEN INTO MUSCLE-BOUND AMAZONS

Wrong! The male hormone testosterone is mainly responsible for muscle building – and women simply don't have very much of it. In fact, training with either free weights or on resistance machines is a great way for women to firm and tone muscles, developing an attractive sculpted appearance as the muscles become more visible beneath their naturally higher levels of body fat. Weight training also boosts the metabolism, helping to burn more calories, and is important to help guard against osteoporosis.

IF YOU STOP EXERCISING, YOUR MUSCLES TURN TO FAT

Wrong! They can't – muscle and fat are completely different substances in the body. How can one turn into the other? This is one of the silliest myths of all!

YOU CAN'T HELP PUTTING ON WEIGHT AS YOU GET OLDER

Wrong! While it's true that from about the age of 30 we lose around one per cent of our strength and cardiovascular fitness per year, that's not an excuse to put your feet up in the expectation of a steady decline into old age. Far from it! Research shows that we can maintain and even improve our physical attributes through exercise as we get older, while there's no reason at all for us to put on weight. That's usually caused by eating the same amount but becoming less active. The solution is simple: do more.

I'LL NEVER LOSE WEIGHT – I COME FROM A FAT FAMILY

Wrong! While we can't change the body type we are born with, we can't blame our genes for making us fat. There's plenty of evidence that fatness runs in families – and the main reason is that they share the same habits of eating too much and exercising too little.

RUNNING IS BAD FOR YOUR KNEES

Wrong! Running is actually good for your knees – and your ankles and hips as well. Scientific studies have shown that moderate amounts of running can help to protect against problems such as osteoarthritis by keeping the major joints of the body strong and mobile. If you don't already have weak ankles and dodgy knees, running in supportive shoes with good posture is very unlikely to start causing problems.

NO PAIN, NO GAIN

Wrong! That discredited phrase comes from the 1980s era of Jane Fonda and 'going for the burn'. Ouch! Exercise is not meant to hurt. Indeed, pain is your body telling you something's wrong – and continuing to exercise through pain could lead to serious injury. You may experience mild discomfort as you begin to exercise regularly, such as muscle soreness and stiffness, but this is your body adapting to the positive changes in your lifestyle and the aches should disappear relatively quickly. If they don't, rest and seek medical advice.

I'M FAT BECAUSE I BURN CALORIES SLOWLY

Wrong! Fatness is not caused by a sluggish metabolism, a notion that was believed for many years. In fact, a study showed that although fat people expend more energy than slim people, they also tend to underestimate how much they eat – by as much as 800 calories per day. That's more than two jam doughnuts. Keeping a diary can help you work out your daily food intake more accurately.

EXERCISE IS BORING

Wrong! Variety is the spice of life – and it's exactly the same with exercise. Anything will become boring if you do it repetitively, mindlessly, day in, day out. The key is to put your mind in gear as well as your body, developing a balanced and varied programme that's fun as well as progressive. If you enjoy a Sunday walk, take a different route. If you do yoga, try a tai chi class. If you like swimming, set yourself a distance or time challenge. Be creative!

HEALTH AND SAFETY

It's always advisable to contact your doctor if you're starting to exercise after a long period of inactivity. It's particularly important to do so if you are pregnant, or if you suffer from any of the following:

- Cardiovascular conditions: previous heart attack or stroke, angina, high/low blood pressure, irregular heartbeat.
- Respiratory conditions: asthma, bronchitis, emphysema, shortness of breath.
- Musculo-skeletal conditions: arthritis, bone disease, ligament or cartilage injury, osteoporosis.
- Blood conditions: haemophilia, leukaemia.
- Other conditions: diabetes, epilepsy, eating disorder, chronic ill health.

Even if you don't suffer from any of these conditions, always take it easy at first. It's great to be enthusiastic, but don't go crazy.

HOW HARD SHOULD I EXERCISE?

It's important to know the intensity at which you're exercising. A simple way to monitor this is the talk test. If you can keep a conversation going while you're active, then you're not exceeding the ability of your aerobic system to provide your working muscles with the oxygen they require.

When you start to gasp, you're going too fast!

Another way to gauge the intensity is to measure your heart rate. First, you need to work out your maximum heart rate (MHR). A good rough guide is to subtract your age from 220.

Now let's work out your resting heart rate. The best time to do this is first thing in the morning. Find the pulse in your carotid (neck) or radial (wrist) artery, using your index and middle fingers (but never the thumb). Count the beats for 15 seconds and multiply by four to get the number of beats per minute. As you begin to exercise regularly, your resting heart rate will decrease – showing that your heart is becoming more efficient. Also, after exercise your heart rate will return to normal more quickly.

The most accurate way to take readings is to buy a heart rate monitor that straps across your chest and feeds information to a digital watch worn on your wrist. A standard model will cost from around £35 and is a very useful investment. Why not treat yourself, or ask for a heart rate monitor as a gift? Most can record info about more than one person. A simple device will keep track of your heart rate and allow you to see how your body reacts to exercise, while a PC-compatible top of the range item will do just about everything, bar the exercise, for you.

Let's now look at the various exercise zones:

- 'Healthy heart zone' is 50–60 per cent of your maximum heart rate (MHR), and is the level at which you should be exercising if you're a beginner, seriously overweight or in cardiac rehabilitation. Steady walking is an ideal fat-burner for anyone looking to exercise in this zone.

- 'Fitness zone' is 60–70 per cent of your MHR, and exercising at this level will produce a significant fat-burning effect. Gentle jogging will get you into this zone.

- 'Training zone' is 70–80 per cent of MHR, and is the level that gives all-round fitness benefits. For example, steady running with your heart rate in this zone will boost your cardiovascular and respiratory system (aerobic fitness) and increase the size and strength of your heart.

- Although it's very unlikely that you will be exercising beyond your training zone, shall we see what lies beyond?

- 'Anaerobic zone' is 80–90 per cent of MHR, and is the level at which top sportspeople improve their 'VO2 max' (the highest amount of oxygen you can consume during exercise) and lactate tolerance (ability to fight the fatigue caused by the build-up of lactic acid in the muscles). This is hard work!

- 'Red-line zone' is 90–100 per cent of MHR, and is as tough as it gets. Even the fittest can only exercise for short periods of time at this level – but in an Olympic 800m final, for example, much of the race will be run in this zone.

The key thing to remember about exercise intensity is that everyone's different. Your age, sex, weight and level of fitness mean your resting and maximum heart rates will be unique to you. However, you can use these figures and an understanding of the exercise zones to help you monitor your progress.

LOVE YOUR BODY!

It can sometimes be hard not to envy the pencil-thin women we see on TV or at the cinema, or the guys with their rippling six-packs on the covers of men's fitness magazines. 'Why, oh why can't I look like that?' we wail. Well, the answer is genetics – they were simply born lucky, with body types that predispose them to slimness or the ability to build muscle.

We all have to work with what we've got – and our challenge is to make the most of whatever that is. One of the very best ways to transform body image is by using our body physically. Exercise helps us to stop viewing our body as an object, as something only to be looked at, and turns it into something we can use as a tool to bolster our self-esteem.

As Sam Murphy puts it in her excellent and inspiring book, *Run for Life* (see overleaf for details): 'What you see in the mirror becomes potential, rather than simply packaging, as you learn to define yourself by what your body does rather than by your appearance.'

Exercise will help you get in touch with your body – perhaps for the first time in many years. You'll start to recognize its little quirks and idiosyncrasies and, as you become more active, begin to explore its gradually changing shape.

Love your body! After all, it's the only one you'll ever have.

TEN INSPIRING BOOKS

The Easy Yoga Workbook by Tara Fraser (Duncan Baird). All the bendy basics in an attractive and user-friendly style.

The Exercise Bible by Joanna Hall (Kyle Cathie). This is a really accessible guide to all-round health, fitness and well-being.

The GI Walking Diet by Joanna Hall (Thorsons). Great advice if you're determined to take at least 10,000 steps a day, plus a great eating plan.

Master the Art of Running by Malcolm Balk and Andrew Shields (Collins & Brown). Don't just run, run well with this intelligent and inspiring guide to good technique.

Master the Art of Swimming by Steven Shaw (Collins & Brown). Instead of seeing swimming as a battle against time and distance, Shaw shows how to swim with economy and grace.

Master the Art of Working Out by Malcolm Balk and Andrew Shields (Collins & Brown). Get the most out of your gym sessions and learn how to work out with ease, efficiency and grace.

Richard's 21st-Century Bicycle Book by Richard Ballantine (Pan). First published in 1972 and constantly updated, this definitive guide ranges from choosing the right bicycle to using it for mountain-biking, commuting and competing, fitness and pleasure.

Run for Life by Sam Murphy (Kyle Cathie). Though aimed at women, this fun and comprehensive guide is a fantastic resource for any would-be runner.

Tai Chi at Home by Paul Crompton (Carroll & Brown). This book has a built-in stand so it's really easy to follow the movements and sequences.

Ultimate Pilates by Dreas Reyneke (Vermilion). A comprehensive manual of Pilates theory and practice by one of the world's best teachers.

The Whartons' Back Book by Jim and Phil Wharton (Rodale). Two of the world's top experts show how we can lead a life free of pain with superb stretching and strengthening routines.

CONTACTS

www.sportengland.org/getactive
Inspiration, information and ideas on how to do more sport and physical activity including links to over 100 sporting organisations' websites and information on how to become a sports volunteer.

www.activeplaces.com
Not sure where to find your nearest swimming pool or golf course? Or looking for a local running club? Thousands of places to play sport and get fit are listed.

INDEX